Breast Sonography Review

A REVIEW FOR THE REGISTRY EXAM

Breast Sonography Review

A REVIEW FOR THE ARDMS BREAST EXAM

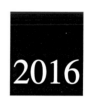

2016

Kathryn A. Gill, MS, RT, RDMS, FSDMS
Institute of Ultrasound Diagnostics
Spanish Fort, Alabama

Special thanks to our prepublication reviewers:

Haven Holstein, BS, RDMS
Lead Sonographer
Florida Hospital
Orlando, Florida

Dana Loveridge Salmons, BS, RT(R), RDMS
Florida Hospital
Orlando, Florida

Davies Publishing, Inc.
32 South Raymond Avenue
Pasadena, California 91105-1935
Phone 626-792-3046
Facsimile 626-792-5308
e-mail info@daviespublishing.com
www.daviespublishing.com

Printed and bound in the United States of America

ISBN 0-941022-75-0

Library of Congress Cataloging-in-Publication Data

Gill, Kathryn A.
  Breast sonography review : a review for the ARDMS breast exam / Kathryn A.
Gill.
    p. ; cm.
  Includes bibliographical references.
  ISBN-13: 978-0-941022-75-0
  ISBN-10: 0-941022-75-7
  1. Breast--Ultrasonic imaging--Examinations, questions, etc. I. Title.
  [DNLM: 1. Ultrasonography, Mammary--Examination Questions. WP 18.2 G475b 2009]
  RG493.5.U47G55 2009
  618.1'907543076--dc22
                                                    2009024703

Preface

THIS MOCK EXAM is a question/answer/reference review of breast sonography for those RDMS candidates who plan to take the ARDMS specialty examination in breast sonography. It is designed as an adjunct to your regular study and as a method to help you determine your strengths and weaknesses so that you can study more effectively. *Breast Sonography Review* covers everything on the current ARDMS exam content outline, which you will find in Part 11 of this book.

Facts about *Breast Sonography Review*:

- It covers the current ARDMS exam outline.

- It focuses exclusively on the Breast specialty exam to ensure thorough coverage of even the smallest subtopic on the exam. (For the Sonography Principles and Instrumentation exam, see *Ultrasound Physics Review for the SPI Exam* by Cindy Owen and James Zagzebski.)

- *Breast Sonography Review* contains nearly 300 questions, many of which are image-based or otherwise illustrated.

- Explanations are clear and conveniently referenced for fact-checking or further study.

- The exam includes Advanced Item Type (AIT) questions that simulate hands-on clinical experience. We have identified the questions in this book that help prepare you for SIC (Semi-Interactive Console) and Hotspot questions.

  SIC questions require the examinee to use a semi-interactive console to correct a problem with the image presented. *Breast Sonography Review* has similar questions that ask what is wrong with an image or how to correct a problem. SIC questions are currently used in the SPI exam. We have included some here to provide bonus Physics coverage.

  Hotspot question items require examinees to indicate the answer to a question by pointing at or marking directly on an image. In *Breast Sonography Review*, similar questions ask examinees to indicate the label on an image that corresponds to the correct answer. Hotspot questions appear on the Breast specialty exam.

- The ARDMS exam outline and contact information for the ARDMS appears in Part 11 at the end of the book.

Breast Sonography Review effectively simulates the content and the experience of taking the exam. Current ARDMS standards call for approximately 170 multiple-choice questions to be answered during a three-hour period. That is, you will have an average time of 1 minute to answer each question. Timing your practice sessions according to the number of questions you need to finish will help you prepare for the pressure experienced by RDMS candidates taking this exam. It also helps to ensure that your practice scores accurately reflect your strengths and weaknesses so that you study more efficiently and with greater purpose in the limited time you can devote to preparation.

ARDMS test results are reported as a "scaled" score that ranges from a minimum of 300 to a maximum of 700. A scaled score of 555 is the passing score (the "passpoint" or "cutoff score" for *all* ARDMS examinations. The scaled score is simply a conversion of the number of correct answers that also, in part, takes into account the difficulty of a particular question. Google or otherwise search for *Angoff scoring method* if you want to learn more about scaled scoring. Suffice it to say that it helps to ensure the fairness of the exams and that in the case of all ARDMS exams 555 is the minimum passing score.

We include below and strongly recommend that you read *Taking and Passing Your Exam*, by Don Ridgway, RVT, who offers useful tips and practical strategies for taking and passing the ARDMS examinations.

Finally, you have not only our best wishes for success, but also our admiration for taking this big and important step in your career.

Kathy Gill

Kathryn A. Gill, MS, RT, RDMS, FSDMS
Spanish Fort, Alabama

Taking and Passing Your Exam

by Don Ridgway, RVT[*]

Preparing for your Exam . . .

Study. And then study some more. Knowing your stuff is the most important factor in your success. Start early, set a regular study schedule, and stick to it. Make your schedule specific so you know exactly what to study on a particular day. Write it down. Establish realistic goals so that you don't build a mountain you can't climb.

As to *what* you study, don't just read aimlessly. Focus your efforts on what you need to know. Rely on a core group of dependable references, referring to others as necessary to firm up your understanding of specific topics. Let the ARDMS exam outlines guide you. And use different but complementary study methods— texts, flashcards, and mock exams—to exercise those neural pathways.

Ease down on studying the week before. Wind down, reduce stress, build confidence, and rest up. Don't cram! And no studying the night before. You had your chance. Watch a movie, relax, go to bed early, and sleep well.

Organize your things the night before. Lay out comfortable clothes (including a sweater or sweatshirt in case the testing center is cold), pencils, your ARDMS test-admission papers, car and house keys, glasses, prescriptions, directions to the test center, and any other personal items you might need. Be prepared!

The Day of Your Exam . . .

Eat lightly. You do not want to fall asleep during the exam. Go easy on the coffee or tea so your bladder doesn't distract you halfway through the exam.

Arrive early. Plan to arrive at the test center early, especially if you haven't been there before. Take directions, including the telephone number of the testing center in case you have to make contact en route. You don't need a wrong-offramp adventure.

---

[*]Don Ridgway is the author of *Introduction to Vascular Scanning: A Guide for the Complete Beginner* and editor of *Vascular Technology Review*. Don is Professor Emeritus at Grossmont College in El Cajon, California.

Be confident. As you wait for the exam to begin, smile, lift both hands, wave them toward yourself, and say, "Bring it on."

During the Exam . . .

Read each question twice before answering. Guess how easy it is to get one word wrong and misunderstand the whole question.

Try to answer the question before looking at the choices. Formulating an answer before peeking at the possibilities minimizes the distractibility of the incorrect answer choices, which in the test-making business are called—guess what!—*distractors*.

Knock off the easy ones first. First answer the questions you feel good about. Then go back for the more difficult items. Next, attack the really tough ones. Taking notes on long or tricky questions often can jog your memory or put the question in new light. For questions you just cannot answer with certainty, eliminate the obviously wrong answer choices and then guess.

Guessing. Passing the exam depends on the number of correct answers you make. Because unanswered questions are counted as *in*correct, it makes sense to guess when all else fails. The ARDMS itself advises that "it is to the candidate's advantage to answer all possible questions." Guessing alone improves your chances of scoring a point from 0 (for an unanswered question) to 25% (for randomly picking one of four possible answers). Eliminating answer choices you know or suspect are wrong further improves your odds of success. By using your knowledge and skill to eliminate two of the four answer choices before guessing, for example, you increase your odds of scoring a point to 50%.

Pace yourself; watch the time. Work methodically and quickly to answer those you know, and make your best guesses at the gnarly ones. Leave no question unanswered.

Don't despair 50 minutes into the exam. At some point you may feel that things just aren't going well. Take 10 seconds to breathe deeply—in for a count of five, out for a count of five. Relax. Recall that you need only about three out of four correct answers to pass. If you've prepared reasonably well, a passing score is attainable even if you feel sweat running down your back.

Taking the Exam on Computer . . .

Some candidates express concern about taking the registry exam on computer. Most folks find this to be pretty easy; some find it off-putting, at least in prospect. But the computerized exams are quite convenient: You can take the exam at your convenience (a far cry from the days of one exam per year), you know whether or not you passed before you leave the testing center (compare that to waiting weeks and even months, as used to be the case), and you can reschedule the exam after 90 days if you happen not to pass the first time (rather than waiting another six months to a year). Another good point: The illustrations are said to be clearer on computer than in the booklets at a Scantron-type exam.

Taking the test by computer is not complicated. The center even gives you a tutorial to be sure you know what you need to do. You sit in a carrel with a computer and answer the multiple-choice questions by pointing and clicking with a mouse. There is a clock on the display letting you know how much time is left. Use it to pace yourself. Scratch paper is available; make liberal use of it.

You can mark questions to return for answering later. A display shows which questions have not been answered so you can return to them. When you have finished, you click on "DONE," and you find out immediately whether you passed.

It's nothing to be afraid of. The principles are the same as those for any exam. Be methodical and keep breathing.

Summary . . .

Preparing for the exam:

- Study
- Use flashcards
- Join a study group
- Wind down a week before
- Don't cram
- Relax!

The day of your exam:

- Eat lightly, avoid coffee
- Arrive early
- Take a sweater
- Be confident!

During the exam:

- Read each question twice
- Answer the question before looking at the answer choices
- Answer the easy ones first
- Guess when necessary
- Don't second-guess your first answers
- Pace yourself
- Don't despair

Taking the exam on computer:

- Just point and click
- Take notes
- Mark and return to the hard questions
- Use the on-screen clock to pace yourself
- Be methodical
- Breathe!

Contents

PART 1

Breast Instrumentation/Technique

System setup

Transducers

Grayscale

Doppler

Physical examination

Mammographic correlation (location and features)

Annotation

Standoff pads

Scan planes

Compressibility

Echo-palpation

Artifacts

Positioning

Indications

1.　Which artifact may cause structures to look deeper than they actually are?

　　A.　Side lobe
　　B.　Shadowing
　　C.　Refraction
　　D.　Propagation speed error
　　E.　Slice thickness

2.　The optimum operating frequency for a broad-bandwidth transducer would be:

　　A.　6 MHz
　　B.　7 MHz
　　C.　8 MHz
　　D.　9 MHz
　　E.　10 MHz

3. In breast sonography, which of the following is NOT significantly affected by the limited field of view when imaging superficial structures?

    A. Contrast resolution
    B. Spatial resolution
    C. Axial resolution
    D. Lateral resolution
    E. Temporal resolution

4. Which of the following affects the actual intensity of the sound utilized for imaging?

    A. TGC
    B. Output power
    C. Overall gain
    D. Dynamic range
    E. Harmonics

    AIT–SIC item.

5. The dynamic range of a display is the:

    A. Number of gray shades
    B. Depth of focal zone
    C. Intensity of sound utilized
    D. Image scale
    E. Output power

    AIT–SIC item.

6. Using color/power Doppler while a patient hums to better delineate a mass is called:

    A. Aliasing
    B. Spectral mirroring
    C. Ring-down
    D. Harmonics
    E. Fremitus

7. A standoff pad thicker than 1 cm is NOT recommended because it will:

    A. Make the skin line look thicker than normal.
    B. Affect the optimal placement of the fixed elevation plane focus.
    C. Compress the mammary layer and make it look fibrotic.
    D. Cause enhancement of echoes in the mammary zone.
    E. Cause decreased penetration and an inability to see the chest wall.

8. Which type of transducer does NOT allow the sonographer to vary the focusing capabilities?

    A. Electronic linear array
    B. Electronic convex array
    C. Annular array

    D. Mechanical sector
    E. Electronic sector

9.   When taking patient history for a breast sonogram, what information from a previous mammogram would NOT be considered relevant?

    A. Symmetry of breasts
    B. Location of a questionable lesion
    C. Size of a questionable lesion
    D. Date and results of a previous mammogram
    E. Name of the radiographer

10.   Image amplitude is affected by:

    A. Power
    B. Overall gain
    C. Time gain compensation (TGC)
    D. A and B
    E. A, B, and C

    AIT–SIC item.

11.   High-frequency transducers used in breast imaging provide excellent resolution of breast tissues but limited:

    A. Focusing options
    B. Gain adjustment
    C. Penetration
    D. Gray scale
    E. Scan lines

12.   When using the 123-ABC method of annotation, "B" would indicate:

    A. Mass is close to the nipple.
    B. Mass is medium shade of gray
    C. Mass is in the mammary zone.
    D. Mass is benign.
    E. Mass requires biopsy.

    AIT–Hotspot item.

13.   In the 123-ABC method of annotation, the numbers denote the:

    A. Distance from nipple
    B. Depth of the mass
    C. Number of masses
    D. Stage of cancer
    E. Sequence of imaging

    AIT–SIC item.

14. Which method of patient positioning is best for evaluating the medial aspect of the breast?

    A. Posterior oblique
    B. Lateral decubitus
    C. Upright
    D. Trendelenburg
    E. Supine

15. The two-handed technique is used to image:

    A. Both breasts at the same time
    B. An extremely large breast
    C. The main breast duct and nipple
    D. Multiple masses within the breast
    E. A palpable mass that is mobile

16. Which of the following transducers would be the best choice for breast imaging?

    A. 5 MHz phased array
    B. 3.5–5 MHz curved linear array
    C. 8 MHz annular array
    D. 10 MHz linear array
    E. 12 MHz mechanical sector

17. Selecting multiple focal zones will:

    A. Decrease frame rate
    B. Increase frame rate
    C. Decrease frequency
    D. Increase frequency
    E. Increase penetration

    AIT–SIC item.

18. When viewing a mammogram, one always sees the marker in the region toward the:

    A. Axilla
    B. Nipple
    C. Medial breast
    D. Top of the film
    E. Bottom of the film

    AIT–Hotspot item.

19. If a breast sonographic image is labeled *Rt. AR 2:00 1A*, the area described is:

    A. In the right axillary region, upper outer quadrant, just under the skin
    B. Radial scan of the right breast, upper outer quadrant, mid breast
    C. Radial scan of the right breast, upper inner quadrant, near the chest wall

D. Antiradial scan of the right breast, upper inner quadrant near the nipple, under the skin

E. Antiradial scan of the right breast, lower inner quadrant, under the skin, near the areola

AIT–Hotspot item.

20. When viewing a mammogram, a mass is marked near the CC marker in the right breast. This will indicate to the sonographer that the mass is located:

A. In the lower outer quadrant
B. In the medial breast
C. In the lateral breast
D. In the upper outer quadrant
E. Near the nipple

AIT–Hotspot item.

21. A transducer that can operate at multiple frequencies is said to have:

A. Broad bandwidth
B. Variable focus
C. Harmonics
D. Multiple transmit zones
E. Dynamic range

22. All of the following statements about high-frequency transducers are true EXCEPT:

A. Axial resolution is increased
B. Lateral resolution is increased
C. Sound travels faster
D. Sound penetration is decreased
E. Best for breast imaging

23. Decreasing depth will:

A. Increase the frequency of sound used
B. Decrease the sound intensity
C. Improve depth penetration
D. Increase the gray scale
E. Increase frame rate

AIT–SIC item.

24. Increasing the overall gain control will:

A. Increase penetration
B. Reduce penetration
C. Cause artifactual echoes
D. Increase gray scale
E. Reduce frame rate

AIT–SIC item.

25. Which of the following allows for better demonstration of small, tortuous vessels?

    A. Power Doppler
    B. Spectral Doppler
    C. Color Flow Doppler
    D. Continuous wave Doppler
    E. Pulsed Doppler

26. Which of the following affect(s) the frame rate?

    A. Number of focal zones
    B. Size of image
    C. Frequency
    D. A and B
    E. A and C

    AIT–SIC item.

27. Ideally, the elevational focus for breast imaging should be fixed at:

    A. 0.5 cm
    B. 1.0 cm
    C. 1.5 cm
    D. 2.0 cm
    E. 2.5 cm

    AIT–SIC item.

28. An increase in the intensity of echoes beneath a structure is called:

    A. Shadowing
    B. Enhancement
    C. Reverberation
    D. Refraction
    E. Reflection

29. Of the following, which would NOT be a good indication for performing a breast sonogram?

    A. Evaluate a mass for microcalcifications
    B. Evaluate a palpable mass
    C. Evaluate a questionable area on mammography
    D. Localize for cyst aspiration
    E. Evaluate a male for gynecomastia

30. When setting the TGC (time gain compensation) control for breast imaging, the following tissue should demonstrate a medium level of gray.

    A. Skin
    B. Fat
    C. Parenchyma

D. Ducts and vessels
E. Muscle

AIT–SIC item.

31. The lactiferous ducts are best seen when scanning:

    A. Radial
    B. Antiradial
    C. Sagittal
    D. Transverse
    E. Coronal

32. The orthogonal view from the longitudinal scan is:

    A. Radial
    B. Antiradial
    C. Transverse
    D. Sagittal
    E. Parallel

33. Adequate penetration of the breast is determined by imaging the:

    A. Lung
    B. Ribs
    C. Deep fascia
    D. Pectoral muscles
    E. Breast parenchyma

34. The arrow is pointing to what kind of artifact?

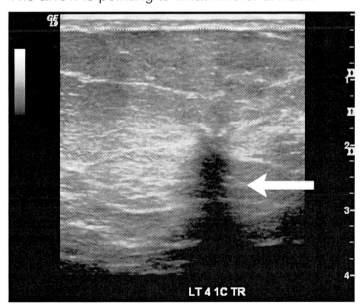

    A. Enhancement
    B. Through transmission
    C. Critical angle refraction
    D. Reverberation

E. Shadow

AIT–Hotspot item.

35. The arrow is pointing to what kind of artifact?

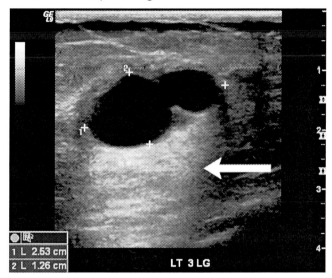

A. Enhancement
B. Ring down
C. Critical angle refraction
D. Reverberation
E. Shadow

AIT–Hotspot item.

36. If a mass is isoechoic with surrounding tissues, what maneuver would accentuate the mass to make it show up better?

A. Add Doppler.
B. Decrease overall gain.
C. Apply harmonics.
D. Try compression.
E. Decrease frequency.

AIT–Hotspot item.

37. Which of the following transducer features would NOT be good for breast imaging?

A. Broad bandwidth
B. High frequency
C. Variable focusing
D. Thin slice thickness
E. Curved linear array format

38. Lateral resolution is best at the:

A. Focal zone
B. Fraunhofer zone

C. Fresnel zone
D. Transmit zone
E. Near zone

39. Which technique would eliminate useful artifacts such as posterior enhancement and shadowing?

    A. Spatial compound imaging
    B. Harmonics imaging
    C. Extended field of view
    D. Dynamic range
    E. Beam focusing

    AIT–SIC item.

40. According to AIUM standards, all of the following information should be indicated on sonographic images of the breast EXCEPT:

    A. Patient's name/ ID #
    B. Patient's age
    C. Patient's social security number
    D. Facility name
    E. Date

41. Which of the following is considered an appropriate annotation method for breast imaging?

    A. Side/quadrant
    B. Clock-face
    C. 123-ABC
    D. All of the above
    E. None of the above

42. Which of the following statements would be FALSE when considering Doppler artifacts?

    A. If the gain and filter settings are too low, it can cause noise.
    B. If the filter setting is too high, it will inhibit the ability to detect low-velocity blood flow.
    C. A PRF/velocity scale that is too low will cause aliasing.
    D. If the Doppler angle is perpendicular to flow, no flow will be detected.
    E. Spectral mirroring causes a duplication of the waveform on the opposite side of baseline.

    AIT–SIC item.

43. Which statement is TRUE for propagation speed error?

    A. If the propagation speed is slower than 1540 m/sec, posterior echoes will be displayed on the sonogram more anterior than they actually are.
    B. If the propagation speed is slower than 1540 m/sec, posterior echoes will be displayed on the sonogram deeper than they actually are.

C. If the propagation speed is faster 1540 m/sec, reflectors will appear closer to the transducer than they actually are.
D. A and B
E. B and C

44. The brightness of echoes on an ultrasound image is affected by all of the following EXCEPT:

A. Overall gain
B. Power output
C. Transducer frequency
D. Dynamic range
E. TGC

AIT–SIC item.

45. Which one of the following steps would NOT be part of the examination preparation?

A. Obtain pertinent clinical information from the patient.
B. Explain the examination to the patient.
C. Present the informed consent to the patient for signature.
D. Review pertinent correlative imaging tests.
E. Know the indication for the exam.

46. The supine oblique position:

A. Evenly distributes the breast tissue
B. Allows better evaluation of the outer breast
C. Places the nipple in the center
D. Minimizes breast thickness for better penetration
E. All of the above

47. Echo palpation is used to:

A. Localize a mass
B. Determine if a mass is compressible or not
C. Determine if a mass is malignant or benign
D. A and B
E. All of the above

48. For general breast scanning, which patient position is considered best?

A. Supine oblique
B. Contralateral posterior oblique
C. Straight supine
D. Upright
E. A and B

49. Of the following, which would NOT be considered a method of annotating the sonographic image?

    A. 123-ABC
    B. Radial/antiradial
    C. Side/quadrant
    D. Clockface
    E. All are acceptable.

PART 2

Normal Anatomy

Ducts (terminal duct lobular unit—TDLU)

Fibrous planes

Skin

Superficial fascia

Mammary zone

Deep fascia

Pectoralis

Ribs

Lymph nodes (internal mammary, axillary, intramammary)

Mammographic versus ultrasonographic appearance

Pregnancy-induced changes

Involutional changes

50. The rapid breast enlargement which begins at puberty is called:

    A. Menarche
    B. Gynecomastia
    C. Thelarche
    D. Hyperplasia
    E. Athelia

51. Breast tissue development is considered functionally complete by:

    A. 20 weeks' gestation
    B. Term
    C. Age 20
    D. Postpartum
    E. Puberty

52. The absence of glandular tissue in the presence of a nipple and areola is called:

    A. Hypoplasia
    B. Athelia
    C. Amastia
    D. Agenesis
    E. Amazia

53. A small rudimentary breast in an adult female is called:

    A. Hypoplasia
    B. Athelia
    C. Amastia
    D. Agenesis
    E. Aplasia

54. When there is glandular breast tissue but no nipple or areola, it is called:

    A. Hypoplasia
    B. Athelia
    C. Amastia
    D. Agenesis
    E. Aplasia

55. The term for accessory, ectopic breast tissue is:

    A. Hyperplastic
    B. Hypoplastic
    C. Mammary ridges
    D. Hypermastic
    E. Supernumerary

56. The most common type of supernumerary breast tissue is:

    A. Polythelia
    B. Polymastia
    C. Hyperthelia
    D. Hypermastia
    E. Multimastia

57. The presence of accessory glandular breast tissue is called:

    A. Polythelia
    B. Polymastia
    C. Hyperthelia
    D. Hypermastia
    E. Multimastia

58. The classification used today for supernumerary breast tissue is:

    A. White's classification
    B. Couinaud's classification
    C. Kajava's classification
    D. Parten's classification
    E. Courvoisier's classification

59. The most common site for polymastia is:

    A. Periumbilical
    B. Mediastinal
    C. Nuchal

    D. Axillary

    E. Facial

60. The mammary ridges are also referred to as the:

    A. Milk lines

    B. Teats

    C. Udders

    D. Nipples

    E. Bosoms

61. The nipple is composed of the following tissue type:

    A. Adipose

    B. Endoplasmic

    C. Areolar

    D. Reticular

    E. Erectile

62. Breast tissue that extends into the axilla is called:

    A. Mastos fascia

    B. Tail of Spence

    C. The colostrum

    D. Premammary zone

    E. Montgomery's zone

63. In the lactating patient, milk production usually begins:

    A. 1 week before delivery

    B. 24–48 hours before delivery

    C. Upon delivery

    D. 2–3 days after delivery

    E. 1 week after delivery

64. The lubricating glands within the areola are called:

    A. Paramammary glands

    B. Montgomery's glands

    C. Glands of Spence

    D. Glands of colostrum

    E. Pectoral glands

65. The darker skin that surrounds the nipple is called the:

    A. Areola

    B. Mammary zone

    C. Superficial fascia

    D. Axilla

    E. Cooper's zone

66. The breast lies directly on the:

    A. Lung
    B. Ribs
    C. Pectoral muscle
    D. Cooper's ligament
    E. Tail of Spence

67. The smallest functional unit of the glandular breast tissue is the:

    A. Lobule
    B. Ductule
    C. Intralobular terminal duct
    D. Extralobular terminal duct
    E. Acini

68. Most breast pathologies originate in the:

    A. Axillary nodes
    B. Areola
    C. Lymph system
    D. Terminal duct lobular unit
    E. Subcutaneous fat

69. The mammary ridges extend from _____ to _____:

    A. Axilla–inguinal region
    B. Axilla–umbilical region
    C. Clavicle–pericostal region
    D. Clavicle–symphysis pubis
    E. Sternum–umbilicus

70. The functional portion of the breast is found within the:

    A. Epidermis
    B. Deep fascia
    C. Lobe
    D. Fat
    E. Nipple

71. The normal skin line should NOT measure more than:

    A. 0.5 mm
    B. 1.0 mm
    C. 1.5 mm
    D. 2.0 mm
    E. 3.0 mm

72. The glandular breast tissue contains all the following structures EXCEPT:

    A. Fat
    B. Acini
    C. Terminal duct lobular units

D. Lactiferous ducts
E. Epithelial/ myoepitheleal cells

73. The primary function of the breast is:

A. Hormone production
B. Excrete sweat
C. Sexual arousal
D. Milk production
E. Infant bonding

74. The number of lobes within each female breast usually range between:

A. 1–5
B. 5–10
C. 10–15
D. 15–20
E. 30–40

75. Which of the following lymph nodes drain 75% of lymph from the breast?

A. Rotter's nodes
B. Axillary nodes
C. Parasternal nodes
D. Supraclavicular nodes
E. Intramammary nodes

76. The lymph nodes located between the pectoral muscles are called:

A. Rotter's nodes
B. Axillary nodes
C. Parasternal nodes
D. Infraclavicular nodes
E. Intrapectoral nodes

AIT–Hotspot item.

77. Of the following statements, which is NOT TRUE of normal intramammary lymph nodes?

A. They are ovoid, have a hyperechoic hilum, and a hypoechoic rim.
B. They are round and have a homogeneous hypoechoic pattern.
C. They usually measure less than 1 cm.
D. They show a vascular pedicle at the hilum
E. Most are found in the posterior upper outer quadrant.

78. The most echogenic tissues within the breast include all of the following EXCEPT:

A. Cooper's ligaments
B. Skin line
C. Ribs

D. Fat

E. Glandular tissue

79. On a mammogram, the most specific indicator of cancer would be:

    A. Nipple retraction
    B. A radiolucent mass
    C. Skin dimpling
    D. Skin thickening
    E. Microcalcifications

80. On a CC mammographic view, a mass that is lateral to the nipple will actually _____ than it appears on the MLO view.

    A. Lie higher
    B. Lie lower
    C. Appear larger
    D. Appear smaller
    E. Appear more superficial

81. The acronym MULD stands for:

    A. Malignant – Undecided – Left – Dominant
    B. Mammo – Upper – Lateral – Dimension
    C. Medial – Up – Lateral – Down
    D. Magnify – Upper – Lactiferous – Ducts
    E. Manage – Under – Legal – Doctor

82. Normal lymph nodes usually measure ≤ 1 cm EXCEPT those found:

    A. Between the pectoral muscles
    B. In the mammary zone
    C. Intercostally
    D. Mediastinal
    E. Axillary

83. The echogenicity of all tissues of the breast is similar to that of:

    A. Glandular parenchyma
    B. Fat
    C. Muscle
    D. Ligaments
    E. Fascia

84. A skin line would be considered abnormally thick if it measured:

    A. 0.5 mm
    B. 1.0 mm
    C. 1.5 mm
    D. 2.0 mm
    E. 3.0 mm

The following illustration applies to questions 85–88.

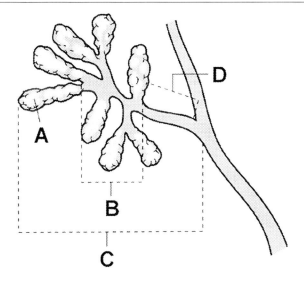

85. In the illustration above, the letter A is pointing to:

   A. Terminal duct lobular unit
   B. Extralobular terminal duct
   C. Intralobular terminal duct
   D. Main lactiferous duct
   E. Ductule

   AIT–Hotspot item.

86. In the illustration above, the letter B is pointing to:

   A. Terminal duct lobular unit
   B. Extralobular terminal duct
   C. Intralobular terminal duct
   D. Main lactiferous duct
   E. Ductule

   AIT–Hotspot item.

87. In the illustration above, the letter C is pointing to:

   A. Terminal duct lobular unit
   B. Extralobular terminal duct
   C. Intralobular terminal duct
   D. Main lactiferous duct
   E. Ductule

   AIT–Hotspot item.

88. In the illustration above, the letter D is pointing to:

   A. Terminal duct lobular unit
   B. Extralobular terminal duct
   C. Intralobular terminal duct

D. Main lactiferous duct

E. Ductule

AIT–Hotspot item.

The following illustration applies to questions 89–96.

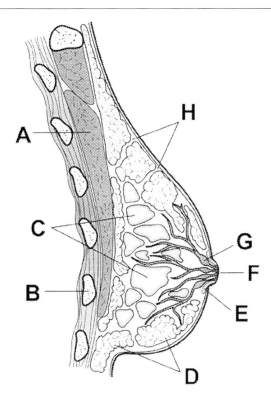

89. In the illustration above, the letter A is pointing to:

A. Cooper's ligament

B. Pectoral muscle

C. Sternum

D. Glandular tissue

E. Lung

AIT–Hotspot item.

90. In the illustration above, the letter B is pointing to:

A. Retromammary lymph node

B. Intramammary lymph node

C. Cooper's ligaments

D. Rib

E. Pectoral muscle

AIT–Hotspot item.

91. In the illustration above, the letter C is pointing to:

A. Fat

B. Glandular tissue
C. Ducts
D. Lymph nodes
E. Terminal duct lobular unit

AIT–Hotspot item.

92. In the illustration above, the letter D is pointing to:

A. Fat
B. Glandular tissue
C. Ducts
D. Lymph nodes
E. Terminal duct lobular unit

AIT–Hotspot item.

93. In the illustration above, the letter E is pointing to:

A. Nipple
B. Duct
C. Areola
D. Cooper's ligament
E. Glandular tissue

AIT–Hotspot item.

94. In the illustration above, the letter F is pointing to:

A. Nipple
B. Duct
C. Areola
D. Cooper's ligament
E. Ductule

AIT–Hotspot item.

95. In the illustration above, the letter G is pointing to:

A. Nipple
B. Duct
C. Areola
D. Cooper's ligament
E. Ductule

AIT–Hotspot item.

96. In the illustration above, the letter H is pointing to:

A. Fat
B. Duct
C. Nodes
D. Cooper's ligament
E. Ductule

AIT–Hotspot item.

97. Which of the following statements is INCORRECT?

    A. Fat exhibits a medium shade of gray.
    B. Fibroglandular tissue is hyperechoic compared to fat.
    C. Muscle is hypoechoic compared to fat.
    D. Cooper's ligaments are isoechoic compared to fat.
    E. Skin is hyperechoic compared to fat.

98. Choose the statement that best describes the order in which breast anatomy is demonstrated sonographically beginning with the skin line.

    A. Skin, fibroglandular tissue, subcutaneous fat, muscle, ribs, lung
    B. Skin, subcutaneous fat, fibroglandular tissue, muscle, ribs, lung
    C. Skin, subcutaneous fat, ribs, fibroglandular tissue, muscle, lung
    D. Skin, ribs, subcutaneous fat, fibroglandular tissue, muscle, lung
    E. Skin, ribs, fibroglandular tissue, fat, lung, muscle

99. Choose the structure(s) included in the terminal duct lobular unit (TDLU).

    A. Acini
    B. Epithelial cells
    C. One terminal duct
    D. One lobule
    E. All of the above

AIT–Hotspot item.

100. Breast atrophy occurs with all of the following conditions EXCEPT:

    A. Breast feeding
    B. Postmenopausal status
    C. Bilateral salpingo-oophorectomy
    D. Fat necrosis
    E. Low fat/high protein diet

101. The best anatomic landmark for localizing parasternal lymph nodes are the:

    A. Subclavian vein and artery
    B. Internal mammary vein and artery
    C. Internal thoracic artery and vein
    D. Axillary artery and vein
    E. None of the above

AIT–Hotspot item.

102. Which of the following make up the skin of the breast?

    A. Epidermis and dermis
    B. Epithelium and myoepithelium
    C. Endoderm and ectoderm
    D. Endoderm and epiderm

E. Ectoderm and epithelium

103. The connective tissues responsible for suspending the breasts are called:

A. Deep fascia
B. Pectoral muscles
C. Lobules
D. Cooper's ligaments
E. Acini

AIT–Hotspot item.

The following image of a normal breast applies to questions 104–108.

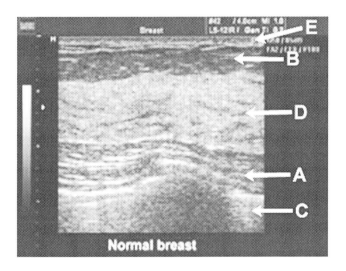

104. In the image above, the letter A corresponds with:

A. Subcutaneous fat
B. Skin
C. Fibroglandular tissue
D. Pleura
E. Pectoral muscle

AIT–Hotspot item.

105. In the image above, the letter B corresponds with:

A. Subcutaneous fat
B. Skin
C. Fibroglandular tissue
D. Pleura
E. Pectoral muscle

AIT–Hotspot item.

106. In the image above, the letter C corresponds with:

A. Subcutaneous fat

B. Skin
C. Fibroglandular tissue
D. Pleura
E. Pectoral muscle

AIT–Hotspot item.

107. In the image above, the letter D corresponds with:

    A. Subcutaneous fat
    B. Skin
    C. Fibroglandular tissue
    D. Pleura
    E. Pectoral muscle

AIT–Hotspot item.

108. In the image above, the letter E corresponds with:

    A. Subcutaneous fat
    B. Skin
    C. Fibroglandular tissue
    D. Pleura
    E. Pectoral muscle

AIT–Hotspot item.

109. The inner portion of breast ducts is lined with:

    A. Basal cells
    B. Epithelial cells
    C. Squamous cells
    D. Transitional cells
    E. Cuboidal cells

110. In this patient who is 6 weeks' postpartum, the arrow points to:

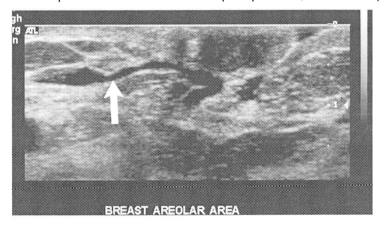

    A. Engorged vessels
    B. Cystic dysplasia
    C. Lactiferous ducts
    D. Arterial ectasia

E. Interlobular fat

AIT–Hotspot item.

The following illustration applies to questions 111–114.

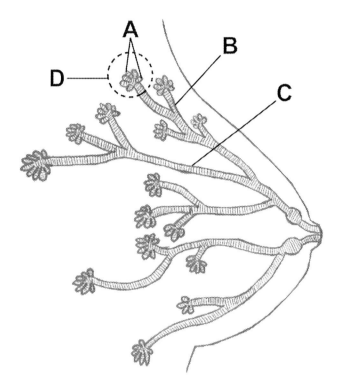

111. In this illustration of breast lobes, letter A corresponds to the:

   A. Acini
   B. Main lactiferous duct
   C. Interlobular terminal duct
   D. Extralobular terminal duct
   E. Terminal duct lobular unit

   AIT–Hotspot item.

112. In this illustration of breast lobes, letter B corresponds to the:

   A. Acini
   B. Main lactiferous duct
   C. Interlobular terminal duct
   D. Extralobular terminal duct
   E. Terminal duct lobular unit

   AIT–Hotspot item.

113. In this illustration of breast lobes, letter C corresponds to the:

   A. Acini

B. Main lactiferous duct
C. Interlobular terminal duct
D. Extralobular terminal duct
E. Terminal duct lobular unit

AIT–Hotspot item.

114. In this illustration of breast lobes, letter D corresponds to the:

    A. Acini
    B. Main lactiferous duct
    C. Interlobular terminal duct
    D. Extralobular terminal duct
    E. Terminal duct lobular unit

    AIT–Hotspot item.

115. On mammography, fat shows a medium gray and is referred to as radiolucent. Which of the following are also considered radiolucent?

    A. Fibroglandular tissue
    B. Solid mass
    C. Pectoral muscle
    D. Serous cyst
    E. Galactocele

116. Which of the following statements is TRUE for mammography?

    A. Detection of calcifications is best seen in dense breast tissues.
    B. Detection of masses is best in the fatty breast.
    C. The standard screening views are the craniocaudal and true lateral views.
    D. Baseline mammograms should begin at age 50.
    E. Side markers are always placed medial to the breast.

117. Which of the following tissues has a water density on mammography?

    A. Fat
    B. Galactocele
    C. Oil-filled cyst
    D. Pectoral muscle
    E. Fibroglandular tissue

118. The artery that supplies oxygenated blood to the inner/medial portion of the breast is the:

    A. Axillary artery
    B. Intercostal artery
    C. Internal thoracic artery
    D. Brachial artery
    E. Subclavian artery

119. Which of the following arteries are NOT included in those supplying blood to the breast?

    A. Axillary artery
    B. Intercostal artery
    C. Internal thoracic artery
    D. Internal mammary artery
    E. Carotid artery

120. The artery that supplies the outer half of the breast is the:

    A. Axillary artery
    B. Intercostals artery
    C. Internal thoracic artery
    D. Internal mammary artery
    E. Carotid artery

121. Which vessel(s) is/are considered a continuation of the axillary artery?

    A. Internal thoracic artery
    B. Intercostal artery
    C. Subclavian artery
    D. Brachial artery
    E. C and D

PART 3

Benign versus Malignant Features

Sharpness of margins

Contour of margins

Border thickness and echogenicity

Shape/orientation

Echogenicity

Heterogeneity

Compressibility

Vascularity

Effects on fibrous planes

Effects on ducts

Calcifications

Lymph nodes

Skin thickening

---

122. All of the following are considered sonographic features of malignancy EXCEPT:

    A. Enhancement
    B. Spiculation
    C. Angular margins
    D. Marked hypoechogenicity
    E. Taller than wide

    AIT–Hotspot item.

123. Of the following findings, which one would NOT be a reliable diagnostic indicator for malignancy?

    A. Posterior enhancement
    B. Hypoechogenicity
    C. Overall acoustic shadowing
    D. Incompressibility
    E. Positive color flow

    AIT–Hotspot item.

124. Which of the following is NOT a sonographic characteristic of a simple cystic mass?

    A. Anechoic
    B. Sharply marginated
    C. Posterior enhancement
    D. Shadowing
    E. Thin walls

    AIT–Hotspot item.

125. When evaluating a mass, you should observe all of the following sonographic features EXCEPT:

    A. Shape
    B. Skin dimpling
    C. Margin definition
    D. Echogenicity
    E. Attenuation

126. If the margins of a mass are thin, defined, and smooth, the indication is that the mass shows signs of:

    A. Host response
    B. Malignancy
    C. Noninvasiveness
    D. Inflammation
    E. Invasiveness

127. A mass that has an uneven distribution of echoes of varying intensities is referred to as:

    A. Cystic
    B. Solid
    C. Complex
    D. Homogeneous
    E. Heterogeneous

128. Which of the following sonographic features would be considered benign?

    A. Thick capsule
    B. Marked hyperechogenicity
    C. Marked hypoechogenicity
    D. Microlobulations
    E. Angular margins

129. If a mass has many very bright echoes, it is referred to as:

    A. Hyperechoic
    B. Hypoechoic
    C. Echogenic
    D. Echopenic
    E. Isoechoic

130. When a malignant tumor infiltrates surrounding tissues, a thick rind of bright echoes can be seen around it. The term for this reaction is called:

  A. Spiculation
  B. Compression
  C. Inflammation
  D. Host response
  E. Ductal extension

  AIT–Hotspot item.

131. Which of the following statements would NOT apply to microcalcifications?

  A. They cast acoustic shadows.
  B. They suggest malignancy.
  C. They measure less than 5 mm in size.
  D. They are not well defined sonographically.
  E. They are best seen on mammogram.

132. A tumor that has grown into several small peripheral ducts is referred to as:

  A. Microlobulation
  B. Branch pattern
  C. Spiculation
  D. Angular
  E. Wider than tall

133. The sign that suggests an invasive malignancy on mammography and sonography is:

  A. Microlobulations
  B. Macrolobulations
  C. Spiculation
  D. Angular margins
  E. Architectural distortion

134. Which benign mass can cause a patient to present with a bloody nipple discharge?

  A. Cyst
  B. Lipoma
  C. Fibroma
  D. Hamartoma
  E. Papilloma

135. When using color Doppler to identify blood flow within a suspicious mass, which maneuver would be most helpful?

  A. Use a high-velocity scale.
  B. Use a high filter.
  C. Increase the transducer pressure over the mass.

D. Make sure the Doppler angle is perpendicular.

E. Use low-flow settings.

AIT–SIC item.

136. Of the following BI-RADS characteristics, which is most indicative of malignancy?

A. Clustered calcifications

B. Enlarging mass

C. Nipple retraction

D. Spiculated irregular border

E. Focal architectural distortion

137. According to BI-RADS classification, Category 2 indicates:

A. Inconclusive

B. Negative

C. Benign finding

D. Probably benign

E. Suspicious abnormality

138. A 17-year-old female suffering from mononucleosis discovers a lump in her right axilla. Because of her strong family history of breast cancer, she begins to worry. Sonography reveals an elliptical hypoechoic mass measuring 3.5 cm with an echogenic central area. The mass is moveable but not painful. The most likely diagnosis would be:

A. Fibroadenoma with macrocalcification

B. Reactive lymph node

C. Metastatic sentinel node

D. Accessory glandular tissue

E. Sebaceous cyst

139. If the long axis of a mass is parallel to the skin line, it means the mass is:

A. Wider than tall

B. Taller than wide

C. Superficial

D. Probably malignant

E. Ductal in origin

140. Which of the following features of a mass would be considered a secondary rather than primary feature?

A. Tumor extension into a duct

B. Orientation

C. Margin regularity

D. Attenuation effects

E. Shape

141. A macrocalcification measures:

    A. < 0.1 mm
    B. < 0.5 mm
    C. < 1.0 mm
    D. > 0.1 mm
    E. ≥ 0.5 mm

142. All of the following causes of skin thickening are benign EXCEPT:

    A. Heart failure
    B. Nephrotic syndrome
    C. Mastitis
    D. Lymphatic obstruction
    E. Irradiation

143. The mass in this image demonstrates:

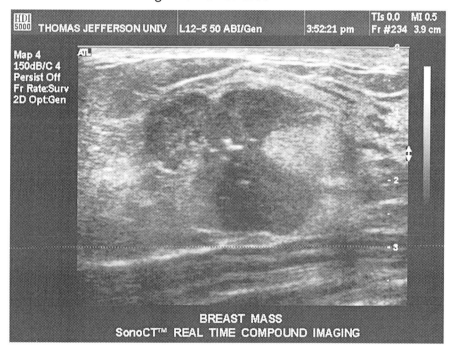

    A. Angular margins
    B. Spiculation
    C. Wider than tall
    D. Microlobulations
    E. Branch pattern

    AIT–Hotspot item.

144. The mass in this image demonstrates:

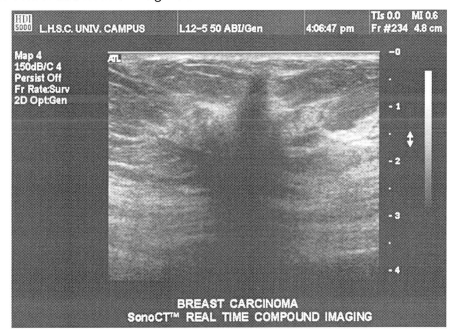

A. Angular margins
B. Spiculation
C. Wider than tall
D. Microlobulations
E. Branch pattern

AIT–Hotspot item.

145. The mass in this image demonstrates:

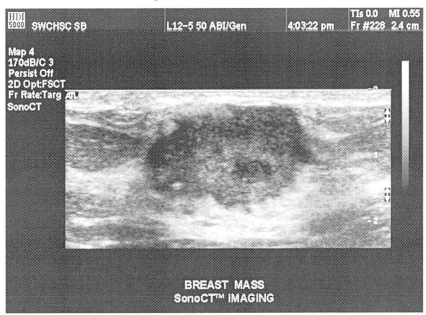

A. Angular margins
B. Spiculation
C. Wider than tall

D. Microlobulations

E. Branch pattern

AIT–Hotspot item.

146. Which of the following sonographic characteristics of malignancy suggest that a tumor is invasive, growing across tissue lines?

A. Spiculation

B. Taller than wide

C. Duct extension

D. Microlobulations

E. Angular margins

AIT–Hotspot item.

147. Which of the following would be considered a benign characteristic?

A. Microlobulations

B. Thick halo

C. Spiculation

D. Hyperechogenicity

E. Indistinct margins

AIT–Hotspot item.

148. All of the following are primary diagnostic features EXCEPT:

A. Shape

B. Lymph node enlargement

C. Margin clarity and regularity

D. Attenuation effects

E. Border thickness

149. All of the following are secondary diagnostic features EXCEPT:

A. Tumor extension

B. Skin changes

C. Homogenicity

D. Interruption of tissue planes

E. Lymph node enlargement

150. All of the following are features of a complex cyst EXCEPT:

A. Fluid debris level

B. Intramural nodule

C. Wall thickening

D. Oval shape

E. Septations

151. Which characteristic is considered a variation of spiculation?

A. Duct extension

B. Microlobulation

C. Disruption of tissue planes

D. Angular margins

E. Thick echogenic halo

152. Which statement does NOT suggest malignancy?

A. A mass has 2–3 macrolobulations.

B. A mass is non-parallel to the chest wall.

C. A mass is markedly hypoechoic.

D. A mass has irregular, ill-defined margins.

E. A mass is incompressible.

153. Which statement would NOT suggest that a mass is benign?

A. The mass is horizontal.

B. The mass is hyperechoic.

C. The mass has microlobulations.

D. The mass has a thin pseudocapsule.

E. The mass shows acoustic enhancement.

154. The mass demonstrated in this image has all of the following characteristics EXCEPT:

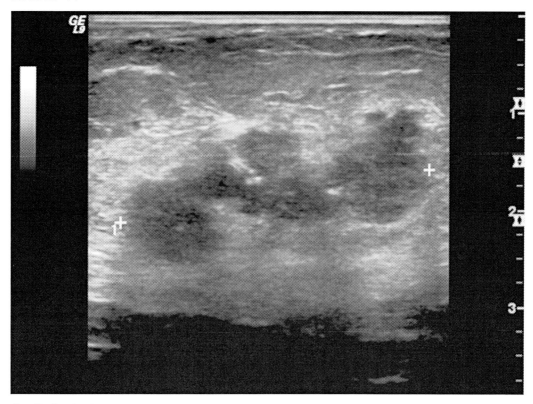

A. Spiculation

B. Microlobulations

C. Markedly hypoechoic

D. Irregular margins

E. Acoustic shadowing

AIT–Hotspot item.

155. Which of the following statements is TRUE?

    A. Benign lesions usually show less internal blood flow than cancers.
    B. Malignant masses are usually wider than tall.
    C. Benign masses usually grow across tissue planes.
    D. Malignant masses are usually markedly hyperechoic.
    E. Benign masses usually demonstrate acoustic shadowing.

156. All of the following conditions can mimic cancer EXCEPT:

    A. Fat necrosis
    B. Radial scar
    C. Sclerosing adenosis
    D. Diabetic mastopathy
    E. Fibroadenoma

157. All of the following conditions can mimic a benign mass EXCEPT:

    A. Medullary carcinoma
    B. Phyllodes tumor
    C. Lymphoma
    D. Metastases
    E. Radiation changes

158. Which of the following statements is FALSE?

    A. Some cancers show posterior enhancement.
    B. Microcalcifications can be seen in benign and malignant tumors.
    C. All cancers show some degree of shadowing.
    D. Abscess and hematomas can disrupt tissue planes.
    E. Cancers usually show more internal blood flow.

159. Regarding nipple discharge, all features listed would be considered benign EXCEPT:

    A. Green, milky discharge
    B. Clear discharge
    C. Expressible only discharge
    D. Multiple duct orifices
    E. Bilateral

160. Regarding lymph nodes, which feature would suggest pathology?

    A. Round shape
    B. Thin capsule
    C. Hypoechoic cortex
    D. Central fatty hilum
    E. Hilar blood flow from single artery

    AIT—Hotspot item.

161. The BI-RADS Classification for Mammography, Ultrasound, and MRI was developed by:

    A. AIUM
    B. ACR
    C. SDMS
    D. AMA
    E. None of the above

PART 4

Specific Lesions—Benign

Cyst

Transmission

Sebaceous cyst

Fibrocystic nodules

Fibroadenoma

Papilloma

Lipoma

Hamartoma

Inflammation and infection

Traumatic changes

Gynecomastia

162. Of the following, which would NOT be considered a complication of breast trauma?

    A. Hematoma
    B. Scarring
    C. Skin thickening
    D. Hamartoma
    E. Fat necrosis

163. A breast mass that is palpable, tender, moveable, compressible, and associated with the menstrual cycle is most likely to be a/an:

    A. Cyst
    B. Abscess
    C. Fibroadenoma
    D. Cancer
    E. Hematoma

164. The most common solid mass seen in women younger than 30 years of age is the:

    A. Medullary carcinoma
    B. Phyllodes tumor
    C. Fibroadenoma
    D. Papilloma
    E. Invasive ductal carcinoma

165. Obstruction of a lactiferous duct in a lactating woman can lead to the development of a/an:

    A. Oil cyst
    B. Galactocele
    C. Sebaceous cyst
    D. Hematoma
    E. Fibroadenoma

166. Mastitis associated with lactation is referred to as:

    A. Granulomatous
    B. Periductal
    C. Puerperal
    D. Ectatic
    E. Apocrine

167. A young patient presents with a bloody nipple discharge from one breast. This is most likely associated with:

    A. Intraductal papilloma
    B. Fibroadenoma
    C. Cystic dysplasia
    D. Cancer
    E. Seroma

168. What is the most common cause of a palpable breast lump in women 35–50 years of age?

    A. Invasive ductal carcinoma
    B. Sebaceous cyst
    C. Intraductal papilloma
    D. Fibroadenoma
    E. Fibrocystic changes

169. Mastitis caused by trauma or infections is referred to as:

    A. Granulomatous mastitis
    B. Periductal mastitis
    C. Puerperal mastitis
    D. Ectatic mastitis
    E. Apocrine mastitis

170. Proliferation of subcutaneous fat and fibroglandular tissue in the male breast is called:

    A. Chronic mammary ectasia
    B. Gynecomastia
    C. Acute fibrocystic dysplasia
    D. Klinefelter syndrome
    E. Puerperal mastitis

171. All of the following are associated with the benign fibroadenoma EXCEPT:

    A. Well-circumscribed
    B. Wider than tall
    C. Fixed
    D. Firm
    E. Solid

172. Of the following which would NOT be associated with fibrocystic changes?

    A. Macrocalcifications
    B. Bloody discharge
    C. Multiple cysts
    D. Hyperechoic glandular tissue
    E. Lumpy, tender breasts

173. Which of the following statements would NOT be true for fibroadenomas?

    A. There is a higher incidence among black females.
    B. Fibroadenomas are benign.
    C. They are common.
    D. They are easily compressible.
    E. Fibroadenomas are stimulated by hormones.

174. A young lactating female presents with a swollen, feverish breast that is extremely tender. Her diagnosis would most likely be:

    A. Hematoma
    B. Phyllodes tumor
    C. Fat necrosis
    D. Cancer
    E. Mastitis

175. All of the following benign pathologies have sonographic features similar to those for malignancy EXCEPT:

    A. Sclerosing adenitis
    B. Fibroadenoma
    C. Fat necrosis
    D. Diabetic mastopathy
    E. Radial scar

176. The sonographic appearance of breast tissue in a lactating patient is best characterized as:

    A. Ground glass
    B. Bag of worms
    C. Cup of milk
    D. Moth-eaten
    E. Swiss cheese

    AIT–Hotspot item.

177. Granulomatous mastitis can be associated with all of the following EXCEPT:

    A. Foreign bodies
    B. Parasitic disease
    C. Tuberculosis
    D. Breast implants
    E. Mondor's disease

178. Of the following masses, which would present as a smooth, well-defined, hyperechoic mass?

    A. Fibroadenoma
    B. Medullary cancer
    C. Abscess
    D. Lipoma
    E. Hamartoma

    AIT–Hotspot item.

179. What mass can develop secondary to traumatic fat necrosis?

    A. Sebaceous cyst
    B. Oil cyst
    C. Simple cyst
    D. Milk cyst
    E. Seroma

180. Thrombophlebitis of the superficial veins of the breast is called:

    A. Mondor's disease
    B. Klinefelter Syndrome
    C. Granulomatous mastitis
    D. Wegener granulomatosis
    E. Giant cell arteritis

181. All of the following are considered acute traumatic breast changes EXCEPT:

    A. Edema
    B. Hematoma
    C. Fat necrosis
    D. Bruising
    E. Skin/tissue retraction

182. A clear fluid-filled mass that may develop following surgery is called a/an:

    A. Cyst
    B. Seroma
    C. Hematoma
    D. Oil cyst
    E. Galactocele

183. Which benign pathology is also referred to as the "swiss cheese disease" because of the classic sonographic appearance of the breast tissue?

   A. Phyllodes tumor
   B. Fibrocystic dysplasia
   C. Juvenile papillomatosis
   D. Fibroadenoma
   E. Mondor's disease

   AIT–Hotspot item.

184. Which of the following would NOT be seen following radiation?

   A. Skin thickening
   B. Interstitial fluid
   C. Fat regeneration
   D. Scar formation
   E. Architectural distortion

185. This patient presented with a palpable breast mass that was tender. Her physician palpated an additional mass. A sonogram was ordered. Based on this finding, the patient most likely has:

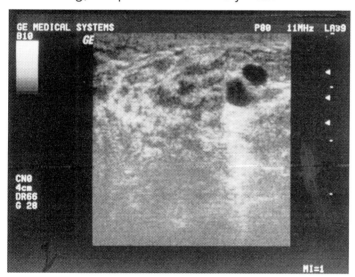

   A. Mastitis
   B. Benign cysts
   C. Fibroadenomas
   D. Fibrocystic dysplasia
   E. Papillomatosis

   AIT–Hotspot item.

186. Which of the following benign masses could be mistaken for a malignant tumor?

   A. Focal fibrosis
   B. Hamartoma
   C. Lipoma

D. Diabetic mastopathy
E. Fibrocystic changes

187. Fibroadenomas are more common among:

A. African Americans
B. Caucasians
C. Hispanics
D. Asians
E. Ethnicity is irrelevant.

PART 5

Specific Lesions—Malignant

DCIS/LCIS

Invasive lesions

Phyllodes

Lymphoma

Metastasis

188. The most common malignant breast tumor is:

   A. Invasive ductal carcinoma
   B. Invasive tubular carcinoma
   C. Medullary carcinoma
   D. Colloid carcinoma
   E. Papillary carcinoma

189. According to the American Cancer Society, 1 out of every ____ women will develop breast cancer:

   A. 2
   B. 4
   C. 6
   D. 8
   E. 10

190. Which of the following is NOT considered a true cancer?

   A. Medullary
   B. Papillary
   C. Ductal carcinoma in situ
   D. Comedo type
   E. Lobular carcinoma in situ

191. The walling off of a tumor with fibrous tissue is the body's attempt to limit invasion. This is referred to as:

   A. Hyperplasia
   B. Neoplasia
   C. Desmoplasia
   D. Hypoplasia
   E. Ectasia

192. All of the following clinical findings are suspicious for breast cancer EXCEPT:

    A. Firm moveable mass
    B. Painless mass
    C. Skin dimpling
    D. Nipple retraction
    E. Bloody nipple discharge

193. Cancers that produce a significant reactive fibrosis around the tumor are referred to as:

    A. Comedo type
    B. Non–comedo type
    C. Granular type
    D. Invasive type
    E. Scirrhous type

194. Which type of breast cancer can mimic a fibroadenoma?

    A. Invasive ductal
    B. Medullary
    C. Colloid
    D. Papillary
    E. Tubular

195. Which tumor is considered the malignant counterpart of the benign fibroadenoma?

    A. Medullary
    B. Colloid
    C. Invasive ductal
    D. Lobular
    E. Phyllodes

196. Of the following primary malignancies, which would be most likely to metastasize to the breast?

    A. Uterine
    B. Ovarian
    C. Melanoma
    D. Gastrointestinal
    E. Renal

197. The most common location for a malignant breast tumor in a female is the:

    A. Subareolar area
    B. Upper outer quadrant
    C. Upper inner quadrant
    D. Lower outer quadrant
    E. Lower inner quadrant

    AIT–Hotspot item.

198. The most common location for a malignant breast tumor in a male is the:

    A. Subareolar area
    B. Upper outer quadrant
    C. Upper inner quadrant
    D. Lower outer quadrant
    E. Lower inner quadrant

    AIT–Hotspot item.

199. Multiple cancer foci within multiple breast quadrants is referred to as:

    A. Multiquad
    B. Multifocal
    C. Multicentric
    D. Bilateral
    E. Multiparous

200. Which of the following is NOT a typical sonographic characteristic of malignant masses?

    A. Shadowing
    B. Markedly hypoechoic
    C. Spiculations
    D. Microlobulations
    E. Wider than tall

201. Which of the following would NOT be considered a risk factor for breast cancer?

    A. Family history
    B. Advanced age
    C. Late menopause
    D. Late menarche
    E. Exogenous estrogen use

202. Which of the following is a noninvasive type of cancer that causes ductal distention filled with a cheese-like material and calcifications?

    A. Comedo type
    B. Non–comedo type
    C. Lobular carcinoma in situ
    D. Phyllodes tumor
    E. Medullary carcinoma

203. An uncommon breast malignancy that develops in younger women, grows rapidly, and has a lower incidence of lymph involvement is called:

    A. Invasive ductal carcinoma
    B. Medullary carcinoma
    C. Sarcoma
    D. Lymphoma
    E. Mucinous carcinoma

204. Another name for the colloid carcinoma is:

    A. Sarcoma
    B. Cystosarcoma phyllodes
    C. Mucinous
    D. Papillomatosis
    E. Metaplasia

205. Multiple tumors within one breast quadrant are referred to as:

    A. Multicentric
    B. Multineoplastic
    C. Multifocal
    D. Multiplastic
    E. Metastatic

206. Which of the following statements is NOT true for inflammatory breast cancer?

    A. It is rare.
    B. Malignant spread is slow.
    C. It gives the breast a "peau d'orange" appearance.
    D. Palpable mass may not be present.
    E. Prognosis is poor.

207. All of the following are sonographic features of a metastatic lymph node EXCEPT:

    A. Smooth oval shape
    B. Enlargement
    C. Asymmetric cortical thickening
    D. Marked hypoechogenicity
    E. Absent hilar fat

208. Which site is the most common for breast cancer to spread via the bloodstream?

    A. Liver
    B. Lung
    C. Brain
    D. Bone
    E. Kidneys

209. Which malignant breast tumor is considered noninvasive?

    A. Medullary
    B. Inflammatory carcinoma
    C. Metastatic breast cancer
    D. Ductal carcinoma in situ
    E. All of the above

210. Which of the following statements is NOT true of lobular carcinoma in situ?

    A. It is the most common noninvasive breast malignancy.
    B. It generally affects premenopausal women.
    C. Mammography and sonography are not usually helpful in detecting a distinct tumor.
    D. It is often multicentric.
    E. It is often bilateral.

211. Which tumor would most likely be found in the postmenopausal patient?

    A. Medullary carcinoma
    B. Papillary carcinoma
    C. Phyllodes tumor
    D. A and B
    E. B and C

212. Which form of ductal carcinoma in situ (DCIS) is most aggressive?

    A. Non–comedo type
    B. Cribriform type
    C. Micropapillary type
    D. Intermediate grade type
    E. Comedo type

213. All of the following are considered histologic categories for breast malignancies EXCEPT:

    A. Tumors of ductal epithelial origin
    B. Tumors of dermal origin
    C. Tumors of lobular origin
    D. Tumors of stromal origin
    E. Metastatic disease

214. The earliest mammographic sign for breast cancer is:

    A. Skin thickening
    B. Nipple retraction
    C. Desmoplasia
    D. Microcalcifications
    E. Ductal dilation

215. Paget's disease is associated with:

    A. Phyllodes tumor
    B. Intracystic papillary carcinoma
    C. Metastatic breast cancer
    D. LCIS
    E. DCIS

216. When primary cancer metastasizes, it usually spreads in the following order:

    A. Bone-lung-brain-liver
    B. Brain-bone-liver-lung
    C. Liver-lung-bone-brain
    D. Lung-liver-brain-bone
    E. Liver-bone-lung-brain

217. Scirrhous type lesions are those that:

    A. Produce a significant reactive fibrosis
    B. Contain clear watery fluid
    C. Contain soft tissue
    D. Are well circumscribed
    E. More likely to be benign

218. All of the following are considered secondary features of invasive breast cancers EXCEPT:

    A. Desmoplasia
    B. Nipple retraction
    C. Retraction of Cooper's ligaments
    D. Spiculation
    E. Skin dimpling

219. Which statement would best describe the colloid carcinoma?

    A. Hard, gritty, and irregular
    B. Soft, lobulated, and compressible
    C. Smooth, hard, and immobile
    D. Hard, lobulated, and moveable
    E. Nonpalpable

220. Which statement(s) is/are true of papillary carcinomas?

    A. Reactive fibrosis is not common.
    B. Shadowing is not usually seen.
    C. They are usually complex in appearance.
    D. A and B
    E. All of the above

221. Which of the following tumors would NOT be considered specific to the breast?

    A. Phyllodes
    B. Lipoma
    C. Medullary carcinoma
    D. Papilloma
    E. Invasive ductal carcinoma

222. A young woman who has recently undergone a lumpectomy and is 6 weeks' post–radiation treatment for DCIS has developed a painful, palpable mass under her incision site. Sonography shows a well-circumscribed hypoechoic mass containing septations and showing some posterior enhancement. Of the following, which is the most likely diagnosis?

    A. Seroma
    B. Hematoma
    C. Mastitis
    D. Oil cyst
    E. Recurrent cancer

223. Of the following carcinomas of the breast, which is considered the rarest?

    A. Colloid
    B. Medullary
    C. Papillary
    D. Inflammatory
    E. Primary lymphoma

224. A lymph node has characteristics associated with metastasis if it is:

    A. Round or lobular
    B. Enlarged
    C. Displaced or absent hilar fat
    D. Is heterogeneous
    E. All of the above

225. Rotter's nodes are included with:

    A. Level I nodes
    B. Level II nodes
    C. Level III nodes
    D. Internal mammary nodes
    E. Supraclavicular nodes

226. A patient presents with erythema of the areola and nipple and itchy nipple discharge with crusting and slight ulceration. These are clinical signs associated with:

    A. Mondor's disease
    B. Diabetic mastopathy
    C. Paget's disease
    D. Cystosarcoma phyllodes
    E. Lymphoma

227. Of the following, which is NOT true of a malignant lymph node?

    A. It will be enlarged.
    B. It shows asymmetrical cortical thickening.
    C. The contour is irregular.

D. It has a single hilar feeding vessel.

E. The hilar fat is displaced or absent.

228. Which primary malignancy, in males, would most likely metastasize to the breast?

A. Liver

B. Lung

C. GI tract

D. Bladder

E. Prostate

229. If a tumor spreads beyond the ductal wall across and into other tissue planes, it is referred to as:

A. Invasive

B. In situ

C. Intralobular

D. Multifocal

E. Multicentric

AIT–Hotspot item.

230. Which of the following would NOT be considered a male risk factor for breast cancer?

A. Advanced age

B. Early andropause

C. Cryptorchidism

D. Family history of breast cancer

E. Radiation exposure

231. Which of the following statements is NOT true for inflammatory breast cancer?

A. It is a common manifestation of invasive ductal carcinoma.

B. Prognosis is poor.

C. It is an uncommon breast cancer.

D. It is a rare sequela to invasive ductal carcinoma.

E. It is a clinical diagnosis.

PART 6

Other

MRI appearance

Ductography

Sentinel node procedure

Histology

Implants

232. Breast imaging that requires the retrograde injection of a radiopaque contrast material into the lactiferous ducts is called:

A. Mammography
B. Scintigraphy
C. PET mammography
D. Galactography
E. Breast MRI

233. Gadolinium is used as a contrast agent for breast imaging with:

A. Mammography
B. Sonography
C. Computerized tomography
D. Magnetic resonance imaging
E. Nuclear medicine

234. When sonography is inconclusive, the following procedure can help differentiate benign from malignant masses:

A. Ductography
B. Galactography
C. Nuclear medicine
D. Magnetic resonance imaging
E. Sentinel node procedure

235. Of the following clinical presentations, which would be best evaluated with ductography?

A. Dense breasts
B. Abnormal nipple discharge
C. Breast asymmetry
D. A and B
E. A and C

236. Breast implant ruptures are best evaluated with:

    A. Mammography
    B. Sonography
    C. Magnetic resonance imaging
    D. Nuclear medicine
    E. Sentinel node procedure

237. The first node to drain lymph from a primary breast cancer is referred to as the:

    A. Primary node
    B. Sentinel node
    C. Terminal node
    D. Axillary node
    E. Lead node

238. With contrast-enhanced MRI, which of the following would be characteristic of invasive breast cancer?

    A. Normal morphologic appearance
    B. Absent rim enhancement
    C. Rapid, moderate to marked tumor enhancement
    D. Slow tumor enhancement
    E. Moderate to marked tumor enhancement

239. Of the following, which is the most common silicone breast implant?

    A. Direct silicone injection
    B. Single lumen, gel-filled
    C. Double lumen, outer saline, and inner silicone
    D. Double lumen, outer silicone, and inner saline
    E. Double lumen saline

240. The sonographic term for the appearance of an intracapsular silicone rupture is:

    A. Stepladder sign
    B. Linguini sign
    C. Teardrop sign
    D. Wavy line sign
    E. Noose sign

    AIT–Hotspot item.

241. The MRI term for the appearance of an intracapsular silicone rupture is:

    A. Stepladder sign
    B. Linguini sign
    C. Teardrop sign

D. Wavy line sign

E. B and D

AIT–Hotspot item.

242. Breast augmentation used for postmastectomy reconstruction is usually placed:

A. Beneath the skin

B. Anterior to the pectoralis muscle

C. Posterior to the pectoralis muscle

D. Anterior to the serratus muscle

E. Posterior to the serratus muscle

243. Scar tissue that often develops around an implant is referred to as:

A. Fibrous capsule

B. Silicone rupture

C. Silicone herniation

D. Capsular contraction

E. Capsular ptosis

244. Which of the following statements is/are true of breast MRI?

A. Benign masses can show contrast enhancement and mimic cancer.

B. It is effective in only 50% of patients with DCIS.

C. It can miss microcalcifications.

D. None of the above.

E. All of the above.

245. MRI features that would be worrisome for nodal metastases would be:

A. Nodal enlargement

B. Enhancement on study with contrast

C. No enhancement on study with contrast

D. A and B

E. A and C

246. An uncollapsed silicone rupture where silicone gets trapped within a peripheral fold is called the:

A. Teardrop sign

B. Noose sign

C. Linguini sign

D. Stepladder sign

E. A and B

AIT–Hotspot item.

247. Ductography involves the utilization of:

A. Mammography

B. Nuclear medicine

C. Magnetic resonance imaging
D. Computerized tomography
E. Sonography

248. Ductography would be contraindicated in the presence of:

A. Mastitis
B. Breast pain
C. Nipple discharge
D. Palpable breast mass
E. Breast augmentation

249. The sentinel node biopsy procedure involves:

A. Mammography
B. Nuclear medicine
C. Computed tomography
D. Magnetic resonance
E. Sonography

250. The microscopic study of tissue is called:

A. Microscopy
B. Pathology
C. Histology
D. Dissection
E. Autopsy

251. Which of the following are is/are considered complications of breast augmentation?

A. Glandular ptosis
B. Autoimmune disorders
C. Infection
D. Retraction
E. All of the above

252. Which location would lower the risk of implant capsular contracture?

A. Submammary
B. Submuscular
C. Subcutaneous
D. Intramammary
E. Prepectoral

AIT–Hotspot item.

253. In this patient with breast implants, what is demonstrated in the right implant?

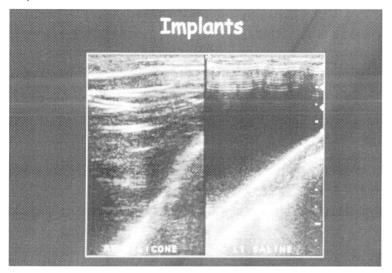

A. Silicone granuloma
B. Stepladder sign
C. Snowstorm appearance
D. Linguini sign
E. Capsular contracture

AIT–Hotspot item.

254. An extracapsular silicone rupture produces the appearance of:

A. Thickened capsule
B. Stepladder
C. Snowstorm
D. Linguini
E. Contracture

AIT–Hotspot item.

255. The most common breast implant in current use is the:

A. Saline-filled single lumen
B. Double lumen–outer saline/inner silicone
C. Double lumen–outer silicone/inner saline
D. Saline inflatable tissue expander
E. Autologous donor tissue

256. Hardening and distortion of an implant due to tightening and constriction of the fibrous capsule is referred to as:

A. Capsular gel bleed
B. Capsular calcification
C. Capsular herniation
D. Capsular rupture
E. Capsular contracture

257. Which of the following would NOT be a normal finding when scanning an augmented breast?

    A. Radial fold
    B. Peripheral fold
    C. Wrinkles
    D. Capsular shell
    E. None of the above

258. Of the following sonographic findings, which is associated with an extracapsular rupture?

    A. Parallel lines
    B. Stepladder sign
    C. Snowstorm sign
    D. Linguini sign
    E. Noose sign

259. A patient presents with subglandular silicone implants. She palpated a mass in her left breast. The sonographic findings suggest:

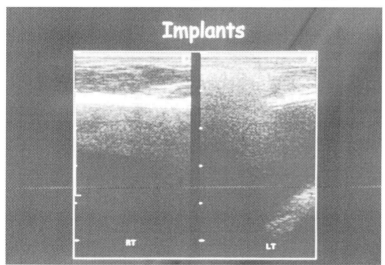

    A. Normal bilateral silicone breast implants
    B. Normal right breast implant, silicone granuloma of the left
    C. Bilateral silicone implant granulomas
    D. Normal bilateral silicone breast implants with cyst in left breast
    E. Normal bilateral silicone breast implants with solid mass in left breast

260. Which imaging modality utilizes non-ionizing technology?

    A. Mammography
    B. Positron emission tomography (PET)
    C. Magnetic resonance imaging (MRI)
    D. Computed tomography (CT)
    E. PET/CT

PART 7

Invasive Procedures

Localizations

Core biopsy

Fine-needle aspiration (FNA)

Mammotomy

Advanced breast biopsy instrumentation (ABBI)

Cyst aspiration

261. All of the following masses would require biopsy or aspiration EXCEPT:

    A. Large painful cyst
    B. Nontender small simple cyst
    C. Solid irregular lesion
    D. Irregular complex mass
    E. Enlarged irregular lymph node

262. Following breast biopsy, patients taking anticoagulants are more likely than others to develop:

    A. Infection
    B. Hematoma
    C. Seroma
    D. Anaphylactic shock
    E. Allergic reaction

263. During an ultrasound-guided breast biopsy, the needle is best imaged when it is _____ to the sound beam.

    A. 45 degrees
    B. 60 degrees
    C. 90 degrees
    D. Perpendicular
    E. Parallel

    AIT–SIC item.

264. Which method used for breast biopsy is the least traumatic for the patient?

    A. Fine-needle aspiration
    B. Spring-loaded automated core biopsy
    C. Vacuum-assisted mammotomy
    D. Advanced breast biopsy instrumentation (ABBI)
    E. Excision

265. The complication of developing a pneumothorax following biopsy is more likely to occur with which method?

    A. Fine-needle aspiration
    B. Spring-loaded automated core biopsy
    C. Vacuum-assisted mammotomy
    D. Advanced breast biopsy instrumentation (ABBI)
    E. Excisional biopsy

266. Undersampling of tissue is more likely with:

    A. Fine-needle aspiration
    B. Spring-loaded automated core biopsy
    C. Vacuum-assisted mammotomy
    D. Advanced breast biopsy instrumentation (ABBI)
    E. Excisional biopsy

267. Which biopsy technique uses a rotating cutting device and vacuum assistance?

    A. Fine-needle aspiration
    B. Mammotomy
    C. Advanced breast biopsy instrumentation (ABBI)
    D. Core biopsy
    E. Excisional biopsy

268. Of the following statements, which is NOT true?

    A. Fine-needle aspiration provides tissues for cytologic analysis.
    B. Cytologic analysis is more conclusive than histologic analysis.
    C. Histologic analysis is more conclusive than cytologic analysis.
    D. Advanced breast biopsy instrumentation (ABBI) can completely excise small lesions.
    E. Mammotomy can completely excise small lesions.

269. Implant rupture would be less likely with:

    A. Fine-needle aspiration
    B. Spring-loaded automated core biopsy
    C. Vacuum-assisted mammotomy
    D. Advanced breast biopsy instrumentation (ABBI)
    E. Large-core biopsy

270. Of the following procedures, which one would be most likely to result in a pseudoaneurysm or arteriovenous fistula?

    A. Fine-needle aspiration biopsy
    B. Spring-loaded automated core biopsy
    C. Vacuum-assisted mammotomy
    D. Advanced breast biopsy instrumentation (ABBI)
    E. Large-core biopsy

271. Of the following procedures, which requires mammographic stereotactic guidance?

    A. Fine-needle aspiration biopsy (FNAB)
    B. Spring-loaded core biopsy
    C. Vacuum-assisted mammotomy
    D. Advanced breast biopsy instrumentation (ABBI)
    E. None of the above

272. Which procedure carries the best chance for tumor localization?

    A. FNAB
    B. Spring-loaded core biopsy
    C. Vacuum-assisted mammotomy
    D. Advanced breast biopsy instrumentation (ABBI)
    E. Large-core biopsy

273. Which of the following statements regarding invasive breast procedures is false?

    A. Interventional procedures can be diagnostic and therapeutic.
    B. Aspirin may be given post procedure for pain and inflammation.
    C. Sonography is often the modality of choice for guidance of invasive procedures.
    D. The most common complication is the development of a hematoma.
    E. Sonographic guidance is more comfortable for the patient and faster than stereotactic x-ray guidance.

274. Which of the techniques listed are used as guidance methods during breast interventional procedures?

    A. Free-hand
    B. Parallel-to-chest
    C. Oblique path
    D. Parallel-to-transducer
    E. All of the above

275. Of the following findings during aspiration, which might indicate additional biopsy or excision?

    A. Bloody tap on aspiration
    B. Septations that inhibit full aspiration
    C. Recurrent cyst formation in short period of time
    D. Thick, impenetrable wall
    E. All of the above

PART 8

Image Gallery

276. What technique is being demonstrated in this color Doppler image of a solid breast lesion?

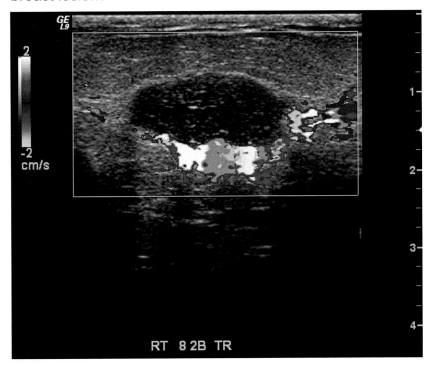

RT 8 2B TR

   A. Compression
   B. Free-hand
   C. Contrast
   D. Fremitus
   E. Power

277. The lesion in the image above was discovered by a 32-year-old female on self-breast exam. It most likely represents:

   A. Sebaceous cyst
   B. Fibroadenoma
   C. Abscess
   D. Carcinoma
   E. Fibrocystic dysplasia

   AIT–Hotspot item.

278. A patient presents 3 weeks' postpartum with breast pain, swelling, and difficulty with lactation. This mass was discovered in the subareolar area. The most likely diagnosis would be:

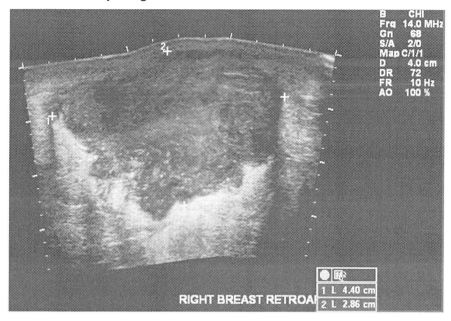

A. Infected cyst
B. Fibroadenoma
C. Fibrocystic dysplasia
D. Abscess
E. Inflammatory carcinoma

AIT–Hotspot item.

279. Patient presents with a small pea-like lump under the skin at the 12:00 o'clock position in the right breast (arrow). Compressibility was demonstrated. This image most likely represents:

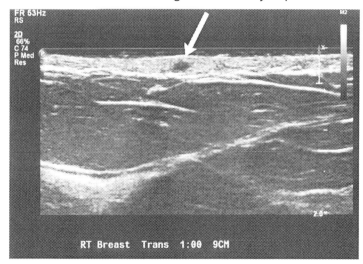

A. Sebaceous cyst
B. Dilated duct

C. Small cancer
D. Lymph node
E. Accessory nipple

AIT–Hotspot item.

The following image applies to questions 280–281.

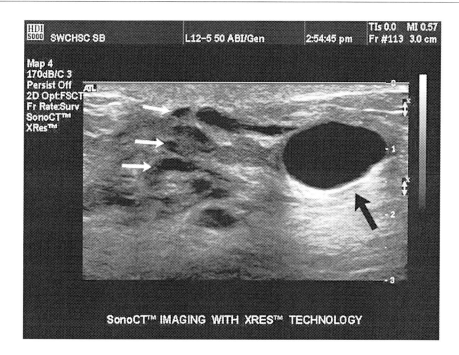

280. In the image above, the mass indicated by the black arrow is most likely:

Λ. Fibroadenoma
B. Malignant tumor
C. Papilloma
D. Abscess
E. Cyst

AIT–Hotspot item.

281. In the image above, the findings indicated by the white arrows were incidental to the exam. They most likely represent:

A. Fibrocystic dysplasia
B. Lymphadenopathy
C. Ductal ectasia
D. Varicoceles
E. Mondor's disease

AIT–Hotspot item.

282. This patient, still within her reproductive years, presents with a bloody nipple discharge. Her sonographic evaluation revealed the findings in this image. The most likely diagnosis would be:

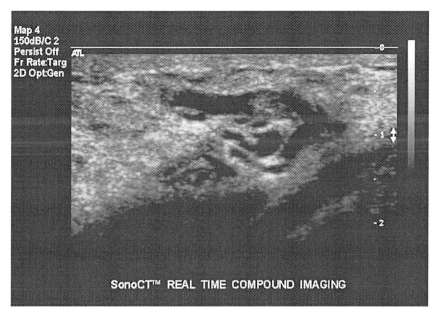

A. Invasive ductal carcinoma
B. Mastitis
C. Mondor's disease
D. Paget's disease
E. Papilloma

AIT–Hotspot item.

283. A 35-year-old female with a family history of breast cancer presents with a palpable lump. Sonography demonstrates what is most likely a:

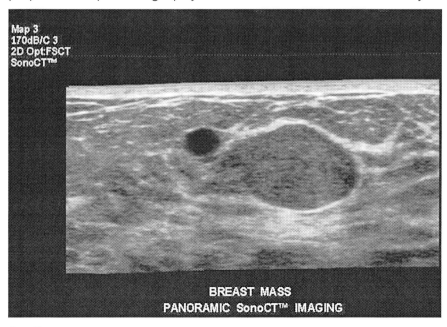

A. Cyst
B. Fibroadenoma
C. Cancer
D. A and B
E. B and C

AIT–Hotspot item.

284. Which malignant characteristic is best demonstrated on this image?

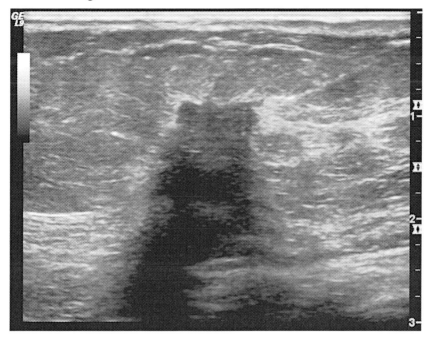

A. Microlobulation
B. Hypoechogenicity
C. Shadowing
D. Wider than tall
E. All of the above

AIT–Hotspot item.

285. This image demonstrates what most likely is a:

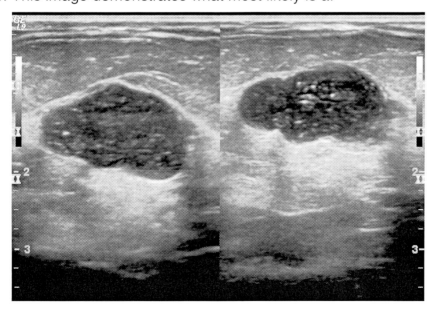

A. Solid mass
B. Complex cyst
C. Fibroadenoma

D. Cancer

E. Lymph node

AIT–Hotspot item.

The following image applies to questions 286–288.

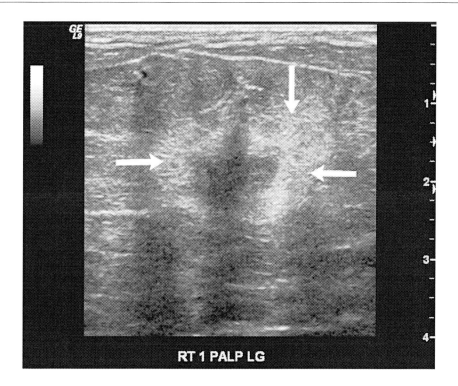

RT 1 PALP LG

286. The arrows in the image above point to:

A. Desmoplasia

B. Posterior enhancement

C. Inflammation

D. Fremitus

E. Thick capsule

AIT–Hotspot item.

287. The mass in the image above demonstrates the following characteristics:

A. Angular margins

B. Hypoechogenicity

C. Shadowing

D. Taller than wide

E. All of the above

AIT–Hotspot item.

288. These sonographic findings would suggest that the mass above is:

A. Benign

B. Malignant

C. Well-defined
D. Complex
E. Pseudomass

289. This mass was proven by biopsy to be malignant. It most likely represents:

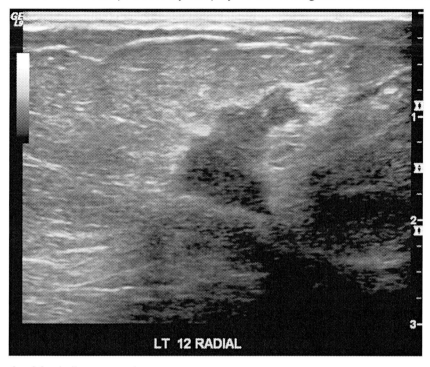

A. Medullary carcinoma
B. Phyllodes tumor
C. Comedo tumor
D. Invasive ductal carcinoma
E. Papilloma

AIT–Hotspot item.

PART 9

Answers, Explanations, and References

BREAST INSTRUMENTATION AND TECHNIQUE

1. D. Propagation speed error.

   Propagation speed error causes structures to look deeper or more superficial than they actually are when the assumed propagation speed (1540 m/sec) is incorrect. The average (and therefore the assumed) propagation speed of ultrasound in human tissue is 1540 meters per second. The greater density and stiffness of some structures—bone, for instance—increase the propagation speed of that tissue, making those structures appear more superficial than they are. Structures of less-than-average density and stiffness—silicone breast implants, for example— have less-than-average propagation speed, making those structures appear to be deeper than they actually are because the sound takes longer than assumed to travel through them. Propagation speed and refraction errors also can distort the displayed shape of a structure.

   ▷Kremkau FW: *Sonography: Principles and Instruments*, 9th edition. St. Louis, MO, Saunders Elsevier, 2016, pp 184–193.

2. E. 10 MHz.

   Both ACR and AIUM indicate that a 10 MHz transducer affords the best penetration of all tissues of the breast. Nevertheless, in clinical practice, transducer selection depends on breast size, density, and location of any mass if present. Many texts now recommend 7.5—13 MHz with optimum elevational plane focus at 1.5 cm to cover it all. The correct answer (E) is the best choice on the exam.

3. E. Temporal resolution.

   Temporal resolution is the ability of a sonographic system to distinguish moving structures or dynamics over time. Temporal resolution is usually not an issue when evaluating the superficial structures of the breast.

4. B. Output power.

   Output power relates to the amplitude of the transmitted voltage and therefore affects the actual intensity of the transmitted sound beam.

5. A. Number of gray shades.

Dynamic range—a measure of the magnitude of signals (echo amplitude) and typically expressed in decibels (dB)—is the ratio of the largest to smallest signal that an ultrasound system can receive, process, and display without distortion. The dynamic range of the ultrasound system can be manipulated by the examiner through TGC and threshold compression settings to increase or decrease contrast resolution. The levels of reflectivity are displayed with the smallest received amplitudes in black and the largest in contrasting white, with the various intermediate levels displayed in shades of gray.

▷Kremkau FW: *Sonography: Principles and Instruments*, 9th edition. St. Louis, MO, Saunders Elsevier, 2016, pp 86–90.

6. E. Fremitus.

When a patient hums, the chest wall and breasts vibrate. Applying color or power Doppler as the patient hums produces a color artifact within normal tissues. Softer breast tissues vibrate more than malignancies and other firm masses, which vibrate less. Firm tissues are therefore visualized as areas of decreased color, even though they may appear isoechoic on the B scan. In a fremitus breast exam, then, a solid mass will be outlined by the color artifact, making it useful in diagnosing breast lesions. (See also The Role of Doppler Technology in the answer to question 135.)

▷Kim MJ, Kim EK, Youk JH, et al: Application of power Doppler vocal fremitus sonography in breast lesions. J Ultrasound Med 25:897–906, 2006.

▷Hagen-Ansert SL, Salsgiver TL, Glenn ME: The breast. In Hagen-Ansert SL: *Textbook of Diagnostic Sonography,* 7th edition. St. Louis, MO, Mosby Elsevier, 2012, p 572.

▷Stavros AT: The breast. In Rumack CM, Wilson SR, Charboneau JW, et al: *Diagnostic Ultrasound*, 4th edition, Volume 1. St. Louis, Mosby Elsevier, 2011, p 813.

7. B. Affect the optimal placement of the fixed elevation plane focus.

When using the optimal 8 MHz transducer, the fixed elevation plane focus is at 1.5 cm; therefore, adding a standoff pad of more than 1 cm would affect that focal zone and resolution.

8. D. Mechanical sector.

9. E. Name of the radiographer.

10. E. (A) Power, (B) Overall gain, and (C) Time gain compensation.

Power applies voltage, thus increasing the overall intensity of the sound. The overall gain increases the brightness of all echoes on the image. TGC adjustments allow the sonographer to increase or decrease the brightness of echoes in specific areas (depths) of the image.

▷Kremkau FW: *Sonography: Principles and Instruments*, 9th edition. St. Louis, MO, Saunders Elsevier, 2016, pp 80–84.

11. C. Penetration.

High frequencies = short wavelengths = less penetration but better resolution.
Low frequencies = long wavelengths = more penetration but decreased resolution.

12. C. Mass is in the mammary zone.

Numbers indicate distance from the nipple. Letters indicate depth in the breast. Measurements are made in cm or mm.

Location within the periphery of the breast is categorized with the numbers 1 through 3. These numbers represent three equal-width rings around the areola, with 1 being central and 3 being peripheral. The depth of the lesion is denoted by the letters A through C: A is the superficial third, B is the middle third (therefore representing the mammary zone), and C is the deep third of the breast. An image of a right breast lesion about 4 cm directly superior to the nipple and 1.5 cm deep that was scanned in a radial plane is described as R 12 2B RAD. A left breast lesion in the UOQ about 6 cm from the nipple and near the chest wall that was scanned in an antiradial plane is described as L 1:30 3C AR.

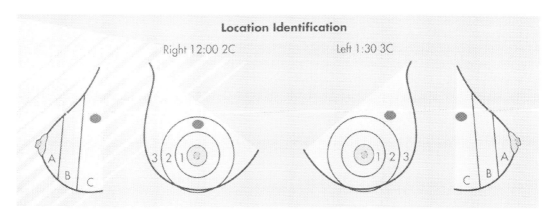

Location Identification

Right 12:00 2C   Left 1:30 3C

▷ Reprinted with permission from Boardman C: Breast. In Gill KA: *Abdominal Ultrasound: A Practitioner's Guide*. St. Louis, Saunders Elsevier, 2001, pp 291–322.

▷Hagen-Ansert SL, Salsgiver TL, Glenn ME: The breast. In Hagen-Ansert SL: *Textbook of Diagnostic Sonography*, 7th edition. St. Louis, MO, Mosby Elsevier, 2012, p 570.

13. A. Distance from the nipple.

See explanation to Answer 12.

14. E. Supine.

When a woman is in the supine position, breast tissue usually falls laterally away from the midline so that the medial breast is flatter and in greater continuity with the chest wall.

15. C. The main breast duct and nipple.

Two hands are required as the nipple is rolled over the sonographer's index finger of one hand while using the other hand to scan along the long axis of the main duct through the nipple.

16. D. 10 MHz linear array.

Linear array transducers allow for imaging perpendicular to the chest wall and provide a larger rectangular field of view, including good visualization in the near field. They are easy to keep in direct contact with the skin, and measurements are reliable because there is no beam divergence along the edges. Linear array transducers offer variable frequency options and narrow and variable focus selections.

17. A. Decrease frame rate.

Frame rate can be affected by changing the number of focal zones, depth of image, and image size.

18. A. Axilla.

19. D. Antiradial scan of the right breast, upper inner quadrant near the nipple, under the skin.

See explanation to Answer 12.

20. C. In the lateral breast.

The mammographic marker CC (craniocaudal) is always placed near the axilla, which is lateral to the breast; therefore, the mass would be located more toward the lateral aspect of the breast.

21. A. Broad bandwidth.

Bandwidth refers to the spectrum of frequencies (high and low) emitted by a transducer.

22. C. Sound travels faster.

For practical purposes, we assume that sound travels through soft tissues at the average speed of 1540 m/sec.

> ▷ Kremkau FW: *Sonography: Principles and Instruments*, 9th edition. St. Louis, MO, Saunders Elsevier, 2016, pp 14–17.

23. E. Increase frame rate.

Frame rate can be affected by changing the number of focal zones, depth of image, and image size.

24. C. Cause artifactual echoes.

    Increasing the overall gain affects the entire image and causes vessels and ducts to fill in with echoes.

25. A. Power Doppler.

    Power Doppler is less angle-dependent and more sensitive to low-flow states. It relies on the number of moving red blood cells more than their velocity. It demonstrates perfusion but provides no information related to direction of flow. (See also The Role of Doppler Technology in the answer to question 135.)

26. D. (A) Number of focal zones and (B) Size of image.

    Frame rate can be affected by changing the number of focal zones, depth of image, and image size.

27. C. 1.5 cm.

28. B. Enhancement.

29. A. Evaluate a mass for microcalcifications.

    Although microcalcifications are readily identified on mammography and an indication of breast cancer, they are too small to resolve sonographically as calcifications.

30. B. Fat.

    All breast tissues are compared to fat since fat should exhibit a mid level shade of gray on sonography.

31. A. Radial.

    Lactiferous ducts converge toward the nipple into a main duct. Radial scanning allows for imaging these duct branches in the long axis.

32. C. Transverse.

    Orthogonal is defined as "perpendicular" or "lying at right angles."

33. D. Pectoral muscles.

    There are three distinct layers of the breast that must be imaged: (1) the subcutaneous layer of skin and fat, (2) the mammary layer of parenchymal tissue, and (3) the retromammary layer containing a thin layer of fat and connective tissue that separates the mammary layer from the pectoral muscles.

34. E. Shadow.

35. A. Enhancement.

Enhancement is the increase in echo strength distal to a structure that only weakly attenuates the ultrasound.

▷ Kremkau FW: *Sonography: Principles and Instruments*, 9th edition. St. Louis, MO, Saunders Elsevier, 2016, pp 194–195.

36. C. Apply harmonics.

Harmonics can actually make isoechoic nodules appear markedly hypoechoic, which can be helpful in differentiating mass from normal tissue.

▷Stavros AT: The breast. In Rumack CM, Wilson SR, Charboneau JW, et al: *Diagnostic Ultrasound*, 4th edition, Volume 1. St. Louis, Mosby Elsevier, 2011, pp 780–781.

37. E. Curved linear array format.

38. A. Focal zone.

39. A. Spatial compound imaging.

40. C. Patient's social security number.

41. D. All of the above.

The breast is divided into four quadrants and labeled like a clock. To describe the location of a lesion or area of concern, the sonographer relates it to the position it would be on a clock (e.g., by noting a cyst at the 2 o'clock position in the right breast). See also explanation to Answer 12.

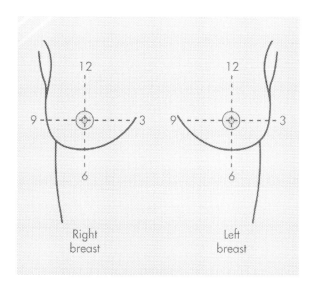

▷Portions reprinted with permission from Boardman C: Breast. In Gill KA: *Abdominal Ultrasound: A Practitioner's Guide*. St. Louis, Saunders Elsevier, 2001, pp 291–322.

▷Hagen-Ansert SL, Salsgiver TL, Glenn ME: The breast. In Hagen-Ansert SL: *Textbook of Diagnostic Sonography,* 7th edition. St. Louis, MO, Mosby Elsevier, 2012, p 569.

42. A. If the gain and filter settings are too low, it can cause noise.

43. E. B and C.

44. C. Transducer frequency.

45. C. Present the informed consent to the patient for signature.

46. E. All of the above.

47. D. A and B

48. E. A and B.

49. E. All are acceptable.

NORMAL ANATOMY

50. C. Thelarche.

51. D. Postpartum.

    Final maturation of female breast lobules occurs with pregnancy and lactation. If pregnancy never occurs, maturation is usually complete 2 years after menarche.

▷Stocksley M, Dixon AM: Breast anatomy and normal ultrasound appearances. In Dixon AM: *Breast Ultrasound: How, Why and When.* Philadelphia, Churchill Livingstone Elsevier, 2007, p 60.

52. E. Amazia.

    Amazia may be congenital or iatrogenic, e.g., the result of radiation therapy, biopsy, or surgery of the developing breast.

53. A. Hypoplasia.

54. B. Athelia.

55. E. Supernumerary.

56. A. Polythelia.

57. B. Polymastia.

58. C. Kajava's classification.

▷Metzker A: *Supernumerary Nipple*. Emedicine. Feb 1, 2007.

59. D. Axillary.

Accessory mammary tissue without areola and nipple is the most common presentation of polymastia and it is most commonly found in the axilla.

▷Stocksley M, Dixon AM: Breast anatomy and normal ultrasound appearances. In Dixon AM: *Breast Ultrasound: How, Why and When.* Philadelphia, Churchill Livingstone Elsevier, 2007, p 61.

60. A. Milk lines.

Also referred to as mammary ridges, the milk lines extend from the axilla to the inguinal regions.

61. E. Erectile

62. B. Tail of Spence.

63. D. 2–3 days after delivery.

▷Shier D, Butler J, Lewis R: *Hole's Anatomy & Physiology*, 13th edition. New York, McGraw Hill, 2012.

64. B. Montgomery's glands.

65. A. Areola.

66. C. Pectoral muscle.

The breasts lie on top of the pectoralis major muscles, with the pectoralis minor muscles lying beneath them. These muscles extend from the 2nd to 6th rib and from the sternum to the axilla.

▷Shier D, Butler J, Lewis R: *Hole's Anatomy & Physiology*, 13th edition. New York, McGraw Hill, 2012.

▷Hagen-Ansert SL, Salsgiver TL, Glenn ME: The breast. In Hagen-Ansert SL: *Textbook of Diagnostic Sonography,* 7th edition. St. Louis, MO, Mosby Elsevier, 2012, pp 550–552.

67. E. Acini.

68. D. Terminal duct lobular unit.

The terminal duct lobular unit (TDLU) is a hormone-sensitive, milk-producing gland that varies in size from 1 to 8 mm in the nonpregnant adult female. At menopause the lobules normally regress in size. In women 55 or more years of age who have breast cancer, however, these lobules remain well-developed.

▷de Paredes ES: *Atlas of Mammography*, 3rd edition. Philadelphia, Lippincott Williams & Wilkins, 2007, p 1.

▷Hagen-Ansert SL, Salsgiver TL, Glenn ME: The breast. In Hagen-Ansert SL: *Textbook of Diagnostic Sonography,* 7th edition. St. Louis, MO, Mosby Elsevier, 2012, pp 550–551.

69. A. Axilla–inguinal region.

▷Dixon AM: *Breast Ultrasound: How, Why and When.* Philadelphia, Churchill Livingstone Elsevier, 2007, p 62.

70. C. Lobe.

71. D. 2.0 mm.

72. A. Fat.

73. D. Milk production.

74. D. 15–20.

75. B. Axillary nodes.

Axillary lymph nodes are typically larger than the others.

76. A. Rotter's nodes.

▷Carr-Hoeffer C: *Breast Ultrasound: A Comprehensive Sonographer's Guide.* Forney, TX, Pegasus Lectures, 2003, p 60.

▷Hagen-Ansert SL, Salsgiver TL, Glenn ME: The breast. In Hagen-Ansert SL: *Textbook of Diagnostic Sonography,* 7th edition. St. Louis, MO, Mosby Elsevier, 2012, p 556.

77. B. They are round and have a homogeneous hypoechoic pattern.

78. D. Fat.

79. E. Microcalcifications.

As many as 80% of breast cancers will show calcifications on histologic examination. These calcifications are usually smaller than 0.2 mm in size.

Imaging characteristics of breast cancer by modality:

Mammography	Sonography	MRI
Spiculation	Spiculation	Rapid, moderate to
Irregular margins	Angular margins	marked tumor
Microlobulations	Microlobulations	enhancement after
Microcalcifications	Calcifications	IV contrast injection
Linear/branching	Branch pattern	
calcifications	Duct extension	

Mass Asymmetric developing density Nipple retraction Skin thickening Enlarged, dense nodes	Taller than wide (nonparallel) Shadowing Marked hypo-echogenicity	Rim enhancement after contrast wash-out

▷Voegeli DR: Mammographic signs of malignancy in breast imaging. In Peters ME, Voegeli DR, Scanlon KA: *Handbook of Breast Imaging*. Churchill-Livingstone, 1989, p 191.

▷Breast cancer: importance of spiculation in computer-aided detection. Radiology 215:703–707, 2000.

▷Stavros AT: The breast. In Rumack CM, Wilson SR, Charboneau JW, et al: *Diagnostic Ultrasound*, 4th edition, Volume 1. St. Louis, Mosby Elsevier, 2011, p 800.

80. B. Lie lower.

81. C. Medial – Up – Lateral – Down.

82. E. Axillary.

83. B. Fat.

84. E. 3.0 mm.

85. E. Ductule.

86. C. Intralobular terminal duct.

87. A. Terminal duct lobular unit.

88. B. Extralobular terminal duct.

89. B. Pectoral muscle.

90. D. Rib.

91. B. Glandular tissue.

92. A. Fat.

93. C. Areola.

94. A. Nipple.

95. B. Duct.

96. D. Cooper's ligament.

97. D. Cooper's ligaments are isoechoic compared to fat.

 Cooper's ligaments are among the most echogenic structures seen within the breast and they may even produce edge shadowing.

98. B. Skin, subcutaneous fat, fibroglandular tissue, muscle, ribs, lung.

99. E. All of the above.

100. A. Breast feeding.

101. C. Internal thoracic artery and vein.

> ▷Madjar H, Mendelson E: *Practice of Breast Ultrasound: Techniques, Findings, and Differential Diagnosis*, 2nd edition. New York, Thieme, 2008.

102. A. Epidermis and dermis.

103. D. Cooper's ligaments.

> ▷Hagen-Ansert SL, Salsgiver TL, Glenn ME: The breast. In Hagen-Ansert SL: *Textbook of Diagnostic Sonography*, 7th edition. St. Louis, MO, Mosby Elsevier, 2012, pp 550–552.

104. E. Pectoral muscle.

105. A. Subcutaneous fat.

106. D. Pleura.

107. C. Fibroglandular tissue.

108. B. Skin.

109. B. Epithelial cells.

110. C. Lactiferous ducts.

111. A. Acini.

112. D. Extralobular terminal duct.

113. B. Main lactiferous duct.

114. E. Terminal duct lobular unit.

115. E. Galactocele.

116. B. Detection of masses is best in the fatty breast.

117. E. Fibroglandular tissue.

On mammography, structures that have a fat density are radiolucent or appear dark (black) on x-ray film. Structures that have a water density are described as radiopaque and appear white on the mammogram. Oil cysts, galactoceles, and fat are radiolucent, while fibroglandular tissue has a water density and may be radiopaque. Pectoral muscles may appear radiopaque, but not always. Therefore, fibroglandular tissue would be the most correct answer choice.

118. C. Internal thoracic artery.

119. E. Carotid artery.

120. A. Axillary artery.

121. E. C and D.

BENIGN VERSUS MALIGNANT FEATURES

122. A. Enhancement.

Malignant features of a solid mass:
- *Spiculation*
- *Angular margins*
- *Taller than wide*
- *Hypoechogenicity*
- *Microcalcification*
- *Duct extension*
- *Branch pattern*
- *Microlobulation*
- *Acoustic shadowing*
- *Disruption of tissue planes*

▷Stavros AT: The breast. In Rumack CM, Wilson SR, Charboneau JW, et al: *Diagnostic Ultrasound*, 4th edition, Volume 1. St. Louis, Mosby Elsevier, 2011, pp 791–801.

123. A. Posterior enhancement.

124. D. Shadowing.

Features of a simple cystic mass include:
- *Round or ovoid shape*
- *Smooth, thin walls*
- *No internal echoes*
- *Posterior enhancement/through transmission*

- *Bilateral edge shadows*

▷Hagen-Ansert SL, Salsgiver TL, Glenn ME: The breast. In
Hagen-Ansert SL: *Textbook of Diagnostic Sonography,* 7th
edition. St. Louis, MO, Mosby Elsevier, 2012, pp 570–572.

Imaging characteristics of benign breast conditions by modality:

Mammography	*Sonography*	*MRI*
Round or ovoid	*Thin capsule*	*Homogeneous low*
Smoothly lobulated	*Smooth borders*	*enhancement with*
Well-defined	*Round or ovoid*	*gradual,*
Presence of fat	*2–3 smooth macrolobulations*	*progressive course*
Macrocalcification	*Enhancement*	*without washout*
	Wider than tall (parallel)	
	Marked hyperechogenicity	
	Homogeneity	
	Well-defined	
	Moveable and compressible	

125. B. Skin dimpling.

Skin dimpling is typically a clinical feature, not a sonographic feature. In cases of extreme skin dimpling, the dimpling can be appreciated sonographically.

126. C. Noninvasiveness.

When a noninvasive mass grows along tissue planes, it will compress the surrounding tissues, creating the appearance of a pseudocapsule, which is thin and can be seen all the way around the mass. An invasive mass would grow across tissue planes, disrupting the capsular echo.

127. E. Heterogeneous.

128. B. Marked hyperechogenicity.

Benign features of a solid mass include:
- *Oval shape/wider than tall*
- *2–3 large, smooth lobulations*
- *Thin pseudocapsule*
- *Marked hyperechogenicity*
- *Homogeneous*
- *Posterior enhancement*

▷Stavros AT: The breast. In Rumack CM, Wilson SR,
Charboneau JW, et al: *Diagnostic Ultrasound,* 4th edition,
Volume 1. St. Louis, Mosby Elsevier, 2011,
pp 801–804.

129. A. Hyperechoic.

130. D. Host response.

The body's typical response to an invasive carcinoma is to wall it off with fibrous tissue in an attempt to limit invasion into surrounding tissues. Other names for this include reactive fibrosis or desmoplasia.

▷Stavros AT: The breast. In Rumack CM, Wilson SR, Charboneau JW, et al: *Diagnostic Ultrasound*, 4th edition, Volume 1. St. Louis, Mosby Elsevier, 2011, p 793.

131. A. They cast acoustic shadows.

132. B. Branch pattern.

133. C. Spiculation.

*Spiculation is the pattern of needle-like lines radiating from a mass. The pattern itself suggests an invasive process and creates irregularities of the border of the mass. The following illustrations, courtesy of Hologic, demonstrate patterns of spiculation found on mammography: **A** Less pronounced radiating lines with absence of central mass (unmarked here because this pattern is less suspicious of malignancy). **B** Less pronounced radiating lines with central mass (marked as suspicious for malignancy). **C** Pronounced radiating lines with absence of central mass (marked as suspicious for malignancy).*

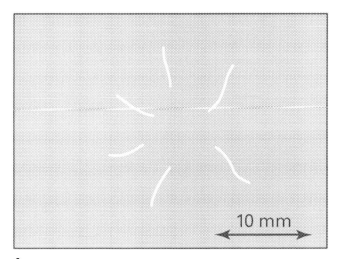

A

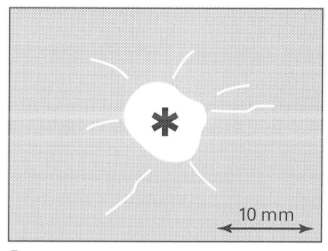

B

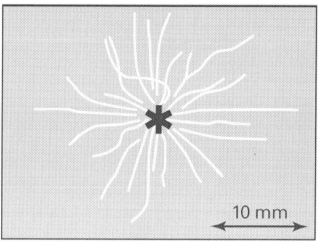

C

Illustrations courtesy of Hologic.

▷Breast cancer: importance of spiculation in computer-aided detection. Radiology 215:703–707, 2000.

▷Stavros AT: The breast. In Rumack CM, Wilson SR, Charboneau JW, et al: *Diagnostic Ultrasound*, 4th edition, Volume 1. St. Louis, Mosby Elsevier, 2011, pp 793–796.

134. E. Papilloma.

135. E. Use low-flow settings.

The Role of Doppler Technology in Breast Sonography

Color flow imaging, power Doppler, and pulsed-wave spectral Doppler are often used in breast imaging. These techniques allow for noninvasive evaluation of blood flow not only within vessels but also in other tissues and masses. Color Doppler is helpful in identifying the small papilloma because it usually is fed by a single vessel. Color Doppler also can be

used to determine if a cyst is infected by showing increased vascularization of the wall. Power Doppler might be employed when the presence of a metastatic node is suspected. Metastatic nodes have very tiny vessels extending to the periphery of the node that feed subcapsular metastatic implants. As noted below, spectral Doppler may also have a role in distinguishing benign from metastatic nodes.

Color Doppler

With color flow imaging (also known as color Doppler), we are able to obtain rapid identification of blood flow within vessels and masses by superimposing a color display over the gray scale image. Flow detection, however, is very angle- and operator-dependent. Unlike gray scale imaging, the blood flow must be parallel to the sound source for optimum visualization. If vasculature is perpendicular to the sound source, no flow will be detected and imaging of these findings could be misleading. If a high flow setting is used, artifactual aliasing will result.

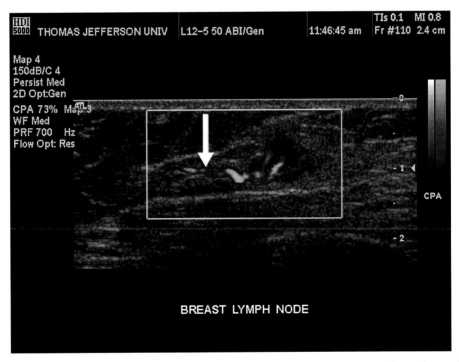

Figure 1. Color Doppler image demonstrating a normal lymph node with a single feeding hilar artery (arrow) and perfusion of the rest of the node.

Power Doppler

Power Doppler, sometimes referred to as power angio, is much less angle-dependent and therefore better at imaging small, tortuous vessels and those with low-flow states. This technique is also good at estimating the total strength of the Doppler shift, but it does not provide information about velocity, flow direction, or turbulence within a vessel. Although power Doppler produces no aliasing artifacts, it is susceptible to motion artifacts. Although power Doppler produces no aliasing artifacts, it is susceptible to motion artifacts.

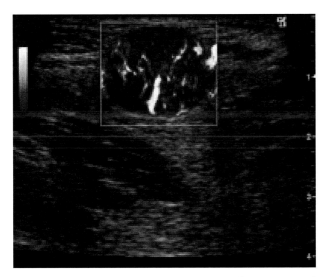

Figure 2. Power Doppler image demonstrating increased vascularity in this malignant lesion.

Pulsed-Wave Spectral Doppler

Pulsed-wave spectral Doppler provides more detailed information about blood flow, such as differentiating arterial from venous flow and laminar from turbulent flow. This technique also allows for measuring mean, peak, and minimal flow velocities and for deriving the pulsatility index (PI) and the resistive index (RI). Although there is some controversy and overlap of information regarding spectral Doppler indices, one example of its utility would be in differentiating an inflammatory or reactive node from a metastatic node. Generally speaking, an inflamed node exhibits a low-resistance waveform and low peak systolic velocities. Velocities from a metastatic node are more likely to be highly resistant with high peak systolic velocities and resistive indices. Like color Doppler, it is angle-dependent, and high velocities can result in aliasing.

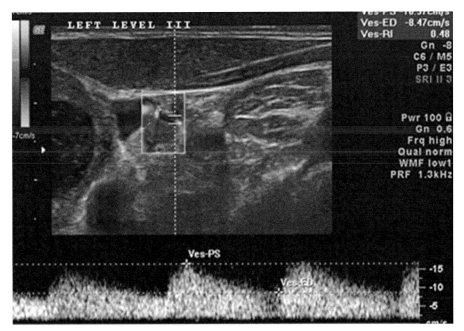

Figure 3. Spectral Doppler waveform revealing low resistance and low peak systolic velocity, which would suggest benign over malignant.

Conclusion

By themselves, these Doppler technologies are not definitively helpful in distinguishing benign from malignant masses because, among other reasons, vascularity is not unique to malignant lesions. The benign fibroadenoma, for example, the most common solid mass in women younger than 30, can be markedly vascularized. Nevertheless, Doppler technology does offer additive information that can help characterize a lesion and refine the diagnosis.

See also the answer to and explanation for question 6 regarding the utility of fremitus in characterizing breast lesions.

▷Stavros AT: The breast. In Rumack CM, Wilson SR, Charboneau JW, et al: *Diagnostic Ultrasound*, 4th edition, Volume 1. St. Louis, Mosby Elsevier, 2011, pp 829–831.

136. D. Spiculated irregular border.

137. C. Benign finding.

   The BI-RADS assessment categories are:

   0: Incomplete
   1: Negative
   2: Benign findings
   3: Probably benign
   4: Suspicious abnormality
   5: Highly suggestive of malignancy
   6: Known biopsy—proven malignancy

138. B. Reactive lymph node.

As part of the body's immune response, lymph nodes enlarge when there is infection or any type of inflammatory process within the body. With mononucleosis, the spleen, which is the largest organ of lymph tissue, can rapidly enlarge along with other lymph nodes throughout the body. The most common sites of lymph node enlargement with mononucleosis are the cervical and axillary regions.

139. A. Wider than tall.

140. A. Tumor extension into a duct.

   Primary features *describe the specific characteristics of the mass, while* **secondary features** *describe the effects of the mass on surrounding tissues. The presence of any malignant feature automatically excludes a mass from a benign classification, and most breast cancers have multiple malignant features.*

   Primary features:
   - *Size*
   - *Shape*
   - *Orientation*
   - *Margin regularity*
   - *Echogenicity*
   - *Homogeneity*
   - *Attenuation effects*

   Secondary features:
   - *Interruption of tissue planes*
   - *Ductal dilatation/tumor extension*
   - *Echogenicity of subcutaneous fat*
   - *Cooper's ligaments: thick-straight-retracted*
   - *Edema/lymphatic dilatation*
   - *Skin changes*
   - *Lymph node enlargement*

   ▷Enion DS, Dixon AM: Benign breast disease. In Dixon AM: *Breast Ultrasound: How, Why and When.* Philadelphia, Churchill Livingstone Elsevier, 2007, pp 139–162.

   ▷Hagen-Ansert SL, Salsgiver TL, Glenn ME: The breast. In Hagen-Ansert SL: *Textbook of Diagnostic Sonography,* 7th edition. St. Louis, MO, Mosby Elsevier, 2012, pp 570–577.

141. E. ≥ 0.5 mm.

142. D. Lymphatic obstruction.

143. A. Angular margins.

144. B. Spiculation.

145. D. Microlobulations.

146. B. Taller than wide.

147. D. Hyperechogenicity.

148. B. Lymph node enlargement.

149. C. Homogenicity.

150. D. Oval shape.

151. E. Thick echogenic halo.

152. A. A mass has 2–3 macrolobulations.

153. C. The mass has microlobulations.

154. A. Spiculation.

155. A. Benign lesions usually show less internal blood flow than cancers.

156. E. Fibroadenoma.

157. E. Radiation changes.

158. C. All cancers show some degree of shadowing.

159. B. Clear discharge.

160. A. Round shape.

Sonographic characteristics of normal versus metastatic lymph nodes:

Normal Lymph Node	Metastatic Lymph Node
Oval with smooth contour	Round and lobulated
Central fatty hilum	Displaced or absent fatty hilum
Symmetry of cortex	Asymmetrical thickening of cortex
Echogenic hilum, hypoechogenic cortex	Heterogeneous, marked hypogenicity
Single hilar feeding vessel	Multiple feeding vessels

161. B. ACR.

BI-RADS (Breast Imaging—Reporting and Data System) was developed, trademarked, and published by the American College of Radiology in collaboration with cooperation from other organizations and committees, including the National Cancer Institute, FDA, AMA, American College of Surgeons, and College of American Pathologists. Conceived as a quality improvement tool and designed to standardize reporting, first for mammography and then for other breast imaging modalities, BI-RADS is published in the form of individual Atlases for mammography, ultrasound, and MRI. The six numerical categories for reporting results are identical for all modalities: 0 = incomplete, 1 = negative, 2 = benign findings, 3 = probably benign, 4 = suspicious abnormality, 5 = highly suggestive of malignancy, and 6 = known biopsy—proven malignancy.

▷www.acr.org

▷D'Orsi CJ, Bassett LW, Berg WA, et al: Breast Imaging Reporting and Data System: ACR BI-RADS-Mammography (ed 4), Reston, VA, American College of Radiology, 2003.

SPECIFIC LESIONS—BENIGN

162. D. Hamartoma.

A hamartoma is an uncommon benign intraglandular tumor made up of normal and dysplastic tissues including fibrous, fatty, and glandular components. Hamartomas may also be called **fibroadenolipomas,** **lipofibroadenomas,** *and* **adenolipomas***.*

▷Salmons D: Breast mass. In Henningsen C, Kuntz K, Youngs D: *Clinical Guide to Sonography: Exercises for Critical Thinking,* 2nd edition. St. Louis, Elsevier Mosby, 2014, pp 329–330.

163. A. Cyst.

Clinical presentations of common breast disorders:

Common Breast Disorders	Clinical Presentation
Fibrocystic changes	Cyclic tenderness, lumpy to palpation. Associated with caffeine and HRT. 30–55 years. May have nipple discharge from several ducts. Symptoms regress with menopause.
Cyst(s)	Asymptomatic or tender palpable nodule, moveable on palpation. 30–50 years.
Fibroadenoma	Hard, firm, very mobile mass on palpation, usually asymptomatic but may be tender. Develops during reproductive

	years. Estrogen influences growth. More common among black females. Regresses with menopause.
Mastitis/abscess	Tender, red, feverish, edematous breast. Skin thickening. May have purulent nipple discharge and tender axillary nodes. Elevated WBC.
Trauma/hematoma	Bruising, edema, skin thickening, tenderness or painful mass.
Papilloma	30–55 years. Subareolar mass. Bloody nipple discharge.
Lipoma	Usually superficial palpable mass that is soft and easily compressible. May be asymptomatic.
Phyllodes	Usually affects postmenopausal patients. Rapidly enlarging mass that is unilateral, nontender, very moveable. Dilated veins seen under skin. May appear lumpy, stretch and discolor skin, and cause ulceration.
Malignant tumor (invasive ductal carcinoma)	Usually postmenopausal. Hard, firm, fixed palpable mass. Skin dimpling, nipple retraction, nipple discharge (clear, bloody, black, creamy), breast asymmetry. May or may not be tender.
Invasive lobular carcinoma	45–55 years. Asymptomatic to palpable nodularity that is ill-defined.

164. C. Fibroadenoma.

165. B. Galactocele.

Benign breast disorders (from most to least common):

Fibrocystic dysplasia
Cyst
Fibroadenoma
Galactocele
Papilloma
Mastitis
Abscess
Mondor's disease
Hematoma
Fat necrosis
Seroma

166. C. Puerperal.

The word "puerperal" denotes a woman who has just given birth to a child and therefore indicates an association with a postpartum incident or

*condition. Mastitis is categorized as **puerperal, periductal**, and **granulomatous**. Of the three, puerperal mastitis is the most common acute type occurring during lactation. If there is a crack in the nipple, bacteria (usually Staphylococcus aureus) enter the duct causing a blockage of the orifice. Milk stasis and bacteria leads to inflammation. The breast becomes edematous, feverish, red, and tender. Some patients present with a purulent nipple discharge and painful axillary lymphadenopathy. On sonography one sees dilated ducts and lymph channels paralleling the skin. There will be edema of the breast parenchyma, interstitial fluid, and skin thickening. Color Doppler reveals hypervascularity of the infected tissues. Abscess formation is a complication of mastitis. It is associated with liquefactive necrosis of the tissues, most of it subareolar in location.*

▷Stavros AT: The breast. In Rumack CM, Wilson SR, Charboneau JW, et al: *Diagnostic Ultrasound*, 4th edition, Volume 1. St. Louis, Mosby Elsevier, 2011, pp 818–819.

▷Hagen-Ansert SL, Salsgiver TL, Glenn ME: The breast. In Hagen-Ansert SL: *Textbook of Diagnostic Sonography,* 7th edition. St. Louis, MO, Mosby Elsevier, 2012, p 576.

167. A. Intraductal papilloma.

168. E. Fibrocystic changes.

169. A. Granulomatous mastitis.

170. B. Gynecomastia.

171. C. Fixed.

172. B. Bloody discharge.

173. D. They are easily compressible.

174. E. Mastitis.

175. B. Fibroadenoma.

Conditions that can mimic breast cancer:

Fat necrosis
Scar tissue
Post radiation changes
Radial scar
Diabetic mastopathy
Sclerosing adenitis
Lymph nodes w/granulomas
Inflammatory fibrous mastopathy

176. A. Ground glass.

177. E. Mondor's disease.

> *Thrombophlebitis of the superficial veins of the anterior chest and breast is called **Mondor's disease**. This is a rare condition of unknown etiology but predisposing factors are thought to include infection, trauma (including recent surgery), a history of a hypercoagulable state, and cancer. There is an inflammatory response to the thrombosis, which surrounds the vein and causes a tender, red, palpable cord-like mass beneath the skin. The onset of pain is sudden, and it may take several months for the vein to recanalize. Recurrences are not uncommon. Mondor's disease may be associated with generalized or localized skin thickening.*

> ▷ Shetty MK, Watson AB. Mondor's disease of the breast. Am J Roentgenol 177:893–896, 2001.

178. D. Lipoma.

179. B. Oil cyst.

180. A. Mondor's disease.

181. E. Skin/tissue retraction.

182. B. Seroma.

183. C. Juvenile papillomatosis.

184. C. Fat regeneration.

185. D. Fibrocystic dysplasia.

186. D. Diabetic mastopathy.

187. A. African Americans.

> *An easy way to remember this fact is to associate the fibrous fibroadenoma to the fibrous fibroid tumor of the uterus. Both are more common among African American females.*

SPECIFIC LESIONS—MALIGNANT

188. A. Invasive ductal carcinoma.

Primary malignant tumors of the breast by type and incidence (%):

Type	Tumor
Invasive (85%)	Invasive ductal carcinoma (60–70%)
	Invasive lobular carcinoma (8–13%)

	Tubular (6–8%)
	Medullary (5%)
	Colloid (2%)
	Papillary (2%)
Noninvasive (15%)	DCIS (10%)
	Intracystic papillary
	Paget's disease
	LCIS

Abbreviations: DCIS = ductal carcinoma in situ, LCIS = lobular carcinoma in situ.

189. D. 8.

190. E. Lobular carcinoma in situ.

191. C. Desmoplasia.

192. A. Firm moveable mass.

Although malignant breast masses are firm and hard, they are usually fixed on palpation due to extension across tissue planes. In contrast, benign solid masses are confined within the tissue plane and moveable.

193. E. Scirrhous type.

194. B. Medullary.

These tumors can grow rapidly and are moveable on physical exam. On sonography they are well marginated, round or oval, and hypoechoic. Both physical and sonographic presentations can be very similar to that of the benign fibroadenoma.

▷ Salmons D: Breast mass. In Henningsen C, Kuntz K, Youngs D: *Clinical Guide to Sonography: Exercises for Critical Thinking*, 2nd edition. St. Louis, Elsevier Mosby, 2014, pp 329–332.

▷Hagen-Ansert SL, Salsgiver TL, Glenn ME: The breast. In Hagen-Ansert SL: *Textbook of Diagnostic Sonography,* 7th edition. St. Louis, MO, Mosby Elsevier, 2012, p 581.

195. E. Phyllodes.

*Microscopically, the **phyllodes tumor** looks very similar to the giant fibroadenoma and can be difficult to differentiate from it. Although usually benign, the phyllodes tumor can have malignant potential. It has been suggested that the term **cystosarcoma phyllodes** be used to denote the malignant form and **giant fibroadenoma** the less aggressive form. Metastasis (10%) depends on the size of the tumor. Large tumors tend to metastasize first to the lungs and then to bone and viscera. Axillary lymph node involvement is usually a late finding.*

▷Salmons D: Breast mass. In Henningsen C, Kuntz K, Youngs D: *Clinical Guide to Sonography: Exercises for Critical*

Thinking, 2nd edition. St. Louis, Elsevier Mosby, 2014, pp 327–328.

196. C. Melanoma.

Most to least common sites of metastasis from primary malignant breast tumor to other site and from other site to breast:

Metastatic from a Breast Primary	Metastatic to Breast from Other Primary*
Axillary lymph nodes	Contralateral breast
Bone	Other primary:
Lung	Melanoma (females)
Brain	Prostate (males)
Liver	Lung
	Ovary
	Sarcoma
	Gastrointestinal
	Hematologic
	Lymphoma (non-Hodgkin's)
	Leukemia

*All of these are rare, accounting for 5% or less.

197. B. Upper outer quadrant.

198. A. Subareolar area.

199. C. Multicentric.

200. E. Wider than tall.

201. D. Late menarche.

Risk factors for breast cancer in women and men:

Women	Men
Postmenopausal	Advanced age
Family history	Exposure to radiation
Early menarche/late menopause	Testicular injury
AMA for first pregnancy	Klinefelter syndrome
Nulliparity/infertility	Cowden's syndrome
High dose radiation exposure	Mumps orchitis
Exogenous estrogen	Family history of breast cancer
Postmenopausal obesity	Chronic diseases

202. A. Comedo type.

Comedo carcinoma tends to be multicentric but confined to medium-sized ducts. Proliferation of the malignant cells will eventually plug the duct(s) and the center portion will necrose.

203. B. Medullary carcinoma.

   Medullary carcinomas are usually large, fleshy masses that are well-circumscribed and moveable. Since they also tend to occur in younger women, they can easily be misdiagnosed clinically as fibroadenomas.

204. C. Mucinous.

205. C. Multifocal.

206. B. Malignant spread is slow.

   Inflammatory breast cancer is a misnomer since it is actually an infiltrating ductal carcinoma with widespread dermal lymphatic invasion that denotes a grave prognosis.

   Typical rate of growth and prognosis of breast tumors:

Type	Fast or Slow	Prognosis
IDC	Variable	Variable to poor
ILC	Variable	More favorable than IDC
Tubular	Slow	Excellent
Medullary	Rapid	Good
Colloid	Slow	Good
Papillary	Slow	Better than IDC NOS
Phyllodes	Rapid	If benign, good; if malignant, variable
Lymphoma	Rapid	Poor

   Abbreviations: IDC = invasive ductal carcinoma, ILC = invasive lobular carcinoma.

   ▷Gilbert-Barness EF: Pathology of the breast. In Peters ME, Voegeli DR, Scanlon KA: *Breast Imaging.* Philadelphia, Churchill Livingstone, 1989, p 13.

   ▷ Salmons D: Breast mass. In Henningsen C, Kuntz K, Youngs D: *Clinical Guide to Sonography: Exercises for Critical Thinking,* 2nd edition. St. Louis, Elsevier Mosby, 2014, pp 330–332.

207. A. Smooth oval shape.

208. D. Bone.

209. D. Ductal carcinoma in situ.

210. A. It is the most common noninvasive breast malignancy.

   Lobular carcinoma in situ *is not considered a true cancer and is often referred to as **lobular hyperplasia** or **lobular neoplasia.** LCIS is a histologic diagnosis and often an incidental finding when a patient has a biopsy for other reasons. The importance of this finding is that the patient is at increased risk for the future development of invasive lobular*

carcinoma. LCIS is multicentric in 70% and bilateral in 30% of patients. Invasive lobular carcinoma is considered the second most common breast cancer.

▷Gilbert-Barness EF: Pathology of the breast. In Peters ME, Voegeli DR, Scanlon KA: *Breast Imaging.* Philadelphia, Churchill Livingstone, 1989, pp 5–6.

▷ Salmons D: Breast mass. In Henningsen C, Kuntz K, Youngs D: *Clinical Guide to Sonography: Exercises for Critical Thinking,* 2nd edition. St. Louis, Elsevier Mosby, 2014, pp 330–331.

211. B. Papillary carcinoma.

212. E. Comedo type.

213. B. Tumors of dermal origin.

Classifications of primary breast cancers include:
- *Lobular*
- *Ductal*
- *Stromal*
- *Phyllodes*
- *Rare/Miscellaneous: apocrine, adenoid cystic, glycogen-rich, metaplastic, squamous, carcinosarcoma.*

▷Gilbert-Barness EF: Pathology of the breast. In Peters ME, Voegli DR, Scanlon KA: *Breast Imaging.* Philadelphia, Churchill Livingstone, 1989, p 6.

▷Salmons D: Breast mass. In Henningsen C, Kuntz K, Youngs D: *Clinical Guide to Sonography: Exercises for Critical Thinking,* 2nd edition. St. Louis, Elsevier Mosby, 2014, pp 330–333.

214. D. Microcalcifications.

215. E. DCIS.

*Other forms of DCIS include **intracystic papillary carcinoma** and **Paget's disease** of the nipple. Most papillary carcinomas are noninvasive, but as they grow they obstruct the duct, forming a cyst. The findings and symptoms are the same as those for benign intracystic papilloma. Paget's disease is an unusual finding associated with (DCIS) ductal carcinoma in situ. Malignant cells migrate along the subareolar duct and extend to the epidermal layer of the nipple and areola. Paget's disease is a clinical rather than radiographic/sonographic diagnosis. The nipple becomes reddened (erythema), ulcerated with eczema-like crustiness and itching. Nipple discharge is common.*

▷Hagen-Ansert SL, Salsgiver TL, Glenn ME: The breast. In Hagen-Ansert SL: *Textbook of Diagnostic Sonography,* 7th edition. St. Louis, MO, Mosby Elsevier, 2012, pp 577–582.

216. A. Bone-lung-brain-liver.

217. A. Produce a significant reactive fibrosis.

218. D. Spiculation.

219. B. Soft, lobulated, and compressible.

220. E. All of the above.

221. B. Lipoma.

> **Lipomas** are simply overgrowth of fatty tissue surrounded by a thin capsule. They are often referred to as **benign fatty tumors**. Lipomas vary in size and are found in many organs of the body, including the liver, kidney, ovary, within the spine, and under the skin, just to mention a few. Lipomas of the breast are usually ovoid in shape, smooth in contour, and may be isoechoic or hyperechoic to the fatty tissues of the breast. They are compressible and may show a small degree of enhancement. It is not uncommon for them to be mixed with other tissues such as muscle/connective tissue (fibromyolipoma) and vessels (angiolipoma or angiomyolipoma).

222. A. Seroma.

223. E. Primary lymphoma.

> Primary lymphoma of the breast accounts for only about 0.12 to 0.53% of all breast malignancies. The prognosis is usually poor, as it is normally widespread.

▷Peters ME: Uncommon malignancies of the breast. In Peters ME, Voegeli DR, Scanlon KA: *Breast Imaging*. Philadelphia, Churchill Livingstone, 1989, p 234.

▷Salmons D: Breast mass. In Henningsen C, Kuntz K, Youngs D: *Clinical Guide to Sonography: Exercises for Critical Thinking*, 2nd edition. St. Louis, Elsevier Mosby, 2014, p 333.

224. E. All of the above.

225. B. Level II nodes.

Surgical classification:

Level I	Inferior axilla	Lateral to pectoralis minor
Level II	Mid axilla	Deep to pectoralis minor
Level III	Superior axilla	Medial to pectoralis minor

▷*Encyclopedia for Surgery: A Guide for Patients and Caregivers*. Internet, Advameg, 2008. [Link: http://www.surgeryencyclopedia.com/A-Ce/Axillary-Dissection.html.]

226. C. Paget's disease.

227. D. It has a single hilar feeding vessel.

228. E. Prostate.

Primary and metastatic breast cancer in men (from most to least common):

Primary	Metastatic to Breast
IDC NOS (85%)	Prostate
DCIS/Paget's disease	Melanoma
Papillary (ductal/intracystic)	Lymphoma
Sarcoma/Lymphoma (4%)	Lung
Other	Bladder

Abbreviations: IDC = invasive ductal carcinoma, NOS = not otherwise specified, DCIS = ductal carcinoma in situ.

229. A. Invasive.

230. B. Early andropause.

231. D. It is a rare sequela to invasive ductal carcinoma.

OTHER

232. D. Galactography.

Galactography—also known as **ductography**—is used to identify the source of abnormal nipple discharge and can be quite helpful when there is no palpable or radiographically detectable mass or abnormality.

233. D. Magnetic resonance imaging.

234. D. Magnetic resonance imaging.

As with any imaging modality, MRI has its advantages and disadvantages. The benefits of breast MRI include the ability to evaluate the young patient with dense breasts. MRI is able to image small lesions within the breast that are sometimes missed on mammography. It is helpful in identifying a primary cancer site in patients with positive axillary lymphadenopathy as well as multifocal, multicentric bilateral disease. In monitoring patients with breast cancer, MRI can differentiate scar tissue from recurrent disease. MRI also can monitor the effects of chemotherapy, making it useful in not only staging disease but also treatment planning. Finally, it is an excellent method for evaluating the breast tissues and implant integrity of patients who have had breast enhancement procedures. Disadvantages include the lack of technology availability, cost, high false-positive findings, and inability to identify microcalcifications.

235. B. Abnormal nipple discharge.

In nonlactating women, fibrocystic dysplasia and benign intraductal papilloma are the most common causes for nipple discharge, which can be serous (fibrocystic) or bloody (papilloma). Galactorrhea and the galactocele are caused by faulty milk production, and the discharge with these conditions contains fat globules. The incidence of nipple discharge associated with malignancy is usually related to the patient's age and the constitution of the discharge. If the woman is young, has no palpable or documented breast mass, and has nonbloody discharge that is bilateral or from multiple ducts, the probability of malignancy is low. A bloody, greenish-black or purulent discharge is always suspicious and requires evaluation regardless of the patient's age.

236. C. Magnetic resonance imaging.

Advantages of MRI:
- *Better imaging of dense breasts*
- *Better for high-risk patients*
- *Better in cases of equivocal mammographic or sonographic findings*
- *Ability to localize primary breast cancer in patient with positive axillary nodes*
- *Good for staging and treatment planning*
- *Ability to evaluate tumor response to chemotherapy*
- *Capable of differentiating scar from tumor recurrence*
- *Improved imaging for implant rupture*

Limitations of MRI:
- *Comparatively expensive*
- *High false-positive rates*
- *Limited effectiveness (only 50% accuracy for ductal carcinoma in situ because microcalcifications can be missed)*
- *Limited availability of facilities with breast coils*
- *Microcalcifications can be missed*

Imaging findings and "signs" in cases of implant complications:

Implant Complication	Sonography	MRI
Capsular contracture	*Thick capsule measuring > 1.5 mm*	
Capsular calcification	*Diffuse shadowing inhabiting visualization*	
Herniation	*Intact implant bulges through capsule*	
Intracapsular rupture	*Stepladder/parallel line sign—multiple linear bands*	*Linguine/wavy line sign*

Uncollapsed rupture	*suspended within silicone gel contained by capsule Keyhole, teardrop, or noose sign—small amount of silicone trapped within a radial fold*	*Keyhole/tear-drop/noose sign*
Extracapsular rupture	*Snowstorm/echogenic noise—hyperechoic echoes projecting beyond capsule with dirty shadowing*	

▷Stavros AT: The breast. In Rumack CM, Wilson SR, Charboneau JW, et al: *Diagnostic Ultrasound*, 4th edition, Volume 1. St. Louis, Mosby Elsevier, 2011, pp 819–824.

▷Dixon AM: *Breast Ultrasound: How, Why and When.* Philadelphia, Churchill Livingstone Elsevier, 2007, p 184.

237. B. Sentinel node.

238. C. Rapid, moderate to marked tumor enhancement.

With MRI imaging, a paramagnetic contrast agent such as gadolinium *is injected intravenously. Malignant tumors, because of their vascularity, show moderate to marked contrast enhancement rather quickly and then wash out. Lesions that show rim enhancement are very suggestive of malignancy. Contrast-enhanced MRI is considered the most sensitive supplemental imaging technique for detecting breast cancer, including primary, nodal, multifocality, and multicentricity.*

▷Stavros AT: The breast. In Rumack CM, Wilson SR, Charboneau JW, et al. *Diagnostic Ultrasound*, 4th edition, Volume 1. St. Louis, Mosby Elsevier, 2011, pp 819–824.

239. B. Single lumen, gel-filled.

240. A. Stepladder sign.

▷Dixon AM: Ultrasound of the augmented breast. In Dixon AM: *Breast Ultrasound: How, Why and When.* Philadelphia, Churchill Livingstone Elsevier, 2007, pp 191–193.

241. E. B and D.

242. C. Posterior to the pectoralis muscle.

Subglandular placement, *also called* **submammary** *and* **prepectoral**, *is commonly used for cosmetic augmentation.* **Subpectoral**, *also called* **retropectoral** *or* **submuscular**, *is more common for postmastectomy reconstruction.*

▷Salmons D: Breast mass. In Henningsen C, Kuntz K, Youngs D: *Clinical Guide to Sonography: Exercises for Critical Thinking*, 2nd edition. St. Louis, Elsevier Mosby, 2014, p 334.

▷Dixon AM: Ultrasound of the augmented breast. In Dixon AM: *Breast Ultrasound: How, Why and When*. Philadelphia, Churchill Livingstone Elsevier, 2007, p 184.

243. A. Fibrous capsule.

244. E. All of the above.

245. D. A and B.

246. E. A and B.

247. A. Mammography.

248. A. Mastitis.

249. B. Nuclear medicine.

*The first node to receive lymph drainage from a primary breast cancer is called the **sentinel node** and is the node at greatest risk for metastasis. This node is typically an axillary node because 75% of lymph from the breast drains to this area. The **sentinel node procedure** involves injecting a blue dye and/or radioisotope, such as technetium-99m labeled as filtered sulfur colloid mixed with saline. The injection is made in front of the breast tumor and/or in the periareolar area. These mapping agents will flow through the lymphatic system and concentrate in the sentinel node, creating a "hot spot" on the nuclear medicine image identifying the sentinel node. The surgeon will then use a scintillation counter or gamma probe to locate the radioactive node for removal and biopsy. The blue dye also will have collected within the node.*

▷Hagen-Ansert SL, Salsgiver TL, Glenn ME: The breast. In Hagen-Ansert SL: *Textbook of Diagnostic Sonography,* 7th edition. St. Louis, MO, Mosby Elsevier, 2012, pp 585–587.

▷Dixon AM: Ultrasound of the augmented breast. In Dixon AM: *Breast Ultrasound: How, Why and When*. Philadelphia, Churchill Livingstone Elsevier, 2007, pp 249–250.

▷Mariani G, Moresco L, Viale G, et al: Radio guided sentinel lymph node biopsy in breast cancer surgery. J Nuclear Med 42:1198–1215, 2001.

250. C. Histology.

251. E. All of the above.

252. B. Submuscular.

253. B. Stepladder sign.

254. C. Snowstorm.

255. A. Saline-filled single lumen.

256. E. Capsular contracture.

*The development of the **fibrous capsule** is one of the more common complications in which a thin rim of scar tissue forms around the implant, usually within weeks of implantation. This scar is the body's normal reaction to a foreign substance.*

***Capsular contracture** occurs as the fibrous capsule gets harder and begins to tighten progressively around the implant. This tightening effect causes the implant to become too rounded, resulting in asymmetry between the breasts. More commonly seen with smooth-shelled subglandular implants, capsular contracture is associated with a fibrous capsule that measures more than 1.5 mm. In some cases, capsular calcifications may develop over time.*

▷Stavros AT: The breast. In Rumack CM, Wilson SR, Charboneau JW, et al: *Diagnostic Ultrasound*, 4th edition, Volume 1. St. Louis, Mosby Elsevier, 2011, pp 819–824.

257. E. None of the above.

258. C. Snowstorm sign.

*An **extracapsular rupture** occurs when there is a break in the implant shell and fibrous capsule allowing silicone to seep into the tissues of the breast, along the chest wall and axilla. The most classic sonographic appearance is the "snowstorm" sign or "echogenic noise." Infiltrated tissues will be hyperechoic and exhibit dirty shadowing.*

▷ Salmons D: Breast mass. In Henningsen C, Kuntz K, Youngs D: *Clinical Guide to Sonography: Exercises for Critical Thinking*, 2nd edition. St. Louis, Elsevier Mosby, 2014, p 334.

▷Stavros AT: The breast. In Rumack CM, Wilson SR, Charboneau JW, et al: *Diagnostic Ultrasound*, 4th edition, Volume 1. St. Louis, Mosby Elsevier, 2011, pp 819–824.

259. B. Normal right breast implant, silicone granuloma of the left.

260. C. Magnetic resonance imaging (MRI).

INVASIVE PROCEDURES

261. B. Nontender small simple cyst.

262. B. Hematoma.

263. D. Perpendicular.

264. A. Fine-needle aspiration.

265. B. Spring-loaded automated core biopsy.

266. A. Fine-needle aspiration.

267. B. Mammotomy.

268. B. Cytologic analysis is more conclusive than histologic analysis.

269. A. Fine-needle aspiration.

270. E. Large-core biopsy.

271. D. Advanced breast biopsy instrumentation (ABBI).

272. D. Advanced breast biopsy instrumentation (ABBI).

Although this technique can completely excise small tumors up to 2 cm in size, it is considered a diagnostic rather than excisional biopsy device by the FDA. Advantages and disadvantages of ABBI are listed below.

Advantages of ABBI:
- *Large-core specimen*
- *Reduces sampling errors*
- *Diagnostic procedure with the ability to excise small lesions*

Disadvantages of ABBI:
- *Limited availability*
- *Expensive*
- *Requires a radiologist and surgeon*
- *Large-specimen removal increases the risk of bleeding/scarring*
- *Removes more normal tissue in path of mass*
- *Requires stitches*
- *If pathology report shows malignancy with unclear margins, surgical excision is still required*

▷Stavros AT: The breast. In Rumack CM, Wilson SR, Charboneau JW, et al: *Diagnostic Ultrasound*, 4th edition, Volume 1. St. Louis, Mosby Elsevier, 2011, pp 833–837.

273. B. Aspirin may be given post procedure for pain and inflammation.

Aspirin and other drugs containing aspirin are not recommended before or after an invasive procedure because aspirin's anticoagulant properties can cause bleeding.

274. E. All of the above.

275. E. All of the above.

IMAGE GALLERY

276. D. Fremitus.

277. B. Fibroadenoma.

278. D. Abscess.

279. A. Sebaceous cyst.

Note the location of the cyst—within the skin itself—and the thin line of communication between the cyst and the surface of the skin, as demonstrated in this magnified view (arrow):

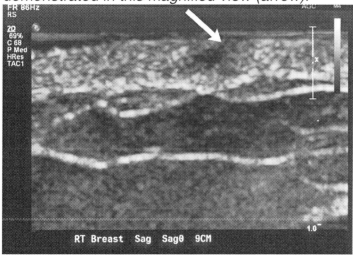

The smooth round or ovoid textbook presentation is often not what is seen clinically. The cyst in this case does not have the perfect definition of a "classic" sebaceous cyst, perhaps because it may no longer be completely intact. The radiologist commented that the line from cyst to skin, the location of the cyst within the skin, and the clinical findings all support the diagnosis of sebaceous cyst. For comparison, here is a "textbook" example of a sebaceous cyst:

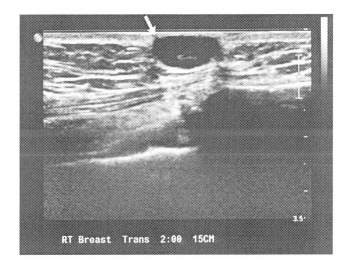

RT Breast Trans 2:00 15CM

The radiologist noted the following: "Palpable nodule reveals a complex hypoechoic circumscribed oval cyst measuring 1.3 x 0.6 x 1.4 cm. The mass is located within the subcutaneous tissues and demonstrates a tract to the skin [arrow]."

Images and commentary courtesy of Fuchsia Loe, MT, RT(M)(CT), RDMS.

280. E. Cyst.

281. C. Ductal ectasia.

282. E. Papilloma.

283. D. A and B.

The fibroadenoma is probably what was initially palpated, with the small adjacent cyst incidentally visualized when sonography was performed.

284. C. Shadowing.

Marked shadowing is demonstrated as a result of the very hard, dense nature of the malignant tumor. The shadowing inhibits visualization of the other borders of tumor, making it ill-defined as well.

285. B. Complex cyst.

Tumors are not compressible, as demonstrated in these "noncompressed" and "compressed" images. A fluid-filled structure will flatten some with compression. Another characteristic demonstrating the fluid nature of the mass is the pronounced posterior enhancement that would not be seen with a cancer or other solid mass. Fibroadenomas occasionally show a small amount of enhancement, but not as pronounced as demonstrated here. Because there are some internal echoes within this cyst, it is best characterized as complex.

286. A. Desmoplasia.

*The body's response to foreign tissue is to wall it off with a fibrous capsule, a process referred to as **host response** or **reactive fibrosis**. This response is often seen with invasive tumors.*

287. E. All of the above.

288. B. Malignant.

289. D. Invasive ductal carcinoma.

The sonographic appearance of medullary carcinoma is similar to that of fibroadenoma and can be mistaken for the same. The phyllodes tumor can be malignant but is often benign and quite large, with areas of necrosis. The comedo tumor is not easily recognized on sonography, and the papilloma is a benign tumor. This mass shows several malignant characteristics, including angular margins, taller than wide, shadowing, desmoplasia, and spiculation.

PART 10

Application for CME Credit

Objectives of this Activity

How To Obtain CME Credit

Applicant Information

Evaluation—You Grade Us!

CME Quiz

This continuing medical educational (CME) activity is approved for 6 hours of credit by the Society of Diagnostic Medical Sonography. This credit may be applied as follows:

- Sonographers and technologists may apply these hours toward the CME requirements of the ARDMS, ARRT, and/or CCI, as well as to the CME requirements of ICAVL for technologists and sonographers in ICAVL-accredited facilities.

- Physicians may apply a certain maximum number of SDMS-approved credit hours toward the CME requirements of the ICAVL for accreditation of diagnostic facilities. (Be sure to confirm current requirements with the pertinent organizations.) Physicians who are registered sonographers or technologists may apply all of these hours toward the CME requirements of the ARDMS, ARRT, and/or CCI. SDMS-approved credit is not applicable toward the AMA Physician's Recognition Award.

If you have any questions about CME requirements that affect you, please contact the responsible organization directly for current information. CME requirements can and sometimes do change.

1. OBJECTIVES OF THE ACTIVITY

Upon completion of this educational activity, you will be able to:

1 Describe and explain the instrumentation and techniques used in breast sonography.
2 Describe and identify the normal anatomy of the breast.
3 Differentiate benign from malignant sonographic findings.
4 Identify and describe specific benign lesions of the breast.
5 Identify and describe specific malignant lesions of the breast.
6 Explain and describe MRI appearance of the breast, ductography, sentinel node procedures, histology, and breast implants.
7 Describe how, when, and why invasive breast procedures are performed.

2. HOW TO OBTAIN CME CREDIT

1 Read and study the book and complete the interactive exercises it contains.
2 Photocopy and then complete this application and CME quiz and the evaluation form below.
3 Make copies of the completed forms for your records and then return the originals (i.e., the photocopied forms with your original writing) to the following address for processing:

> Send us your application, CME answer sheet, evaluation form, and payment by:
>
> **Mail:**
>
> **Davies Publishing, Inc.**
> **Attn: CME Coordinator**
> **32 South Raymond Avenue, Suite 4**
> **Pasadena, California 91105-1935**
>
> **Fax:**
>
> **626-792-5308**
> Pay by credit card number.

3. APPLICANT INFORMATION

Name _____   Birth date _____

Current credentials _____

Home Address _____

City/State/Zip _____

Telephone _____   Email address _____

ARDMS # _____   ARRT # _____   CCI # _____   SDMS # _____

Check Enclosed ☐

Credit Card # _____   Exp. Date _____   3- or 4-digit code: _____

☐ I purchased the book myself. ☐ I borrowed the book.

Signature certifying your completion of the activity and authorizing payment:

_____

NOTE: The original purchaser of this CME activity is entitled to submit this CME application for an administrative fee of $39.50. Please enclose a check payable to Davies Publishing Inc. with your application or a 16-digit credit card number and expiration date. Others may also submit applications for CME credits by completing the activity as explained above and enclosing an administrative fee of $49.50. The CME administrative fee helps to defray the cost of processing, evaluating, and maintaining a record of your application and the credit you earn. Fees may change without notice. For the current fee, call us at 626.792.3046, e-mail us at **cme@DaviesPublishing.com**, or write to us at the aforementioned address. We will be happy to help!

4. ANSWER SHEET

Circle the correct answer below and return this sheet together with the application information and evaluation form to Davies Publishing Inc. or fax to 626-792-5308.

1. A B C D E	21. A B C D E	41. A B C D E
2. A B C D E	22. A B C D E	42. A B C D E
3. A B C D E	23. A B C D E	43. A B C D E
4. A B C D E	24. A B C D E	44. A B C D E
5. A B C D E	25. A B C D E	45. A B C D E
6. A B C D E	26. A B C D E	46. A B C D E
7. A B C D E	27. A B C D E	47. A B C D E
8. A B C D E	28. A B C D E	48. A B C D E
9. A B C D E	29. A B C D E	49. A B C D E
10. A B C D E	30. A B C D E	50. A B C D E
11. A B C D E	31. A B C D E	51. A B C D E
12. A B C D E	32. A B C D E	52. A B C D E
13. A B C D E	33. A B C D E	53. A B C D E
14. A B C D E	34. A B C D E	54. A B C D E
15. A B C D E	35. A B C D E	55. A B C D E
16. A B C D E	36. A B C D E	56. A B C D E
17. A B C D E	37. A B C D E	57. A B C D E
18. A B C D E	38. A B C D E	58. A B C D E
19. A B C D E	39. A B C D E	59. A B C D E
20. A B C D E	40. A B C D E	60. A B C D E

5. Evaluation—You Grade Us!

Please let us know what you think of *Breast Sonography Review*. Participating in this quality survey is a requirement for CME applicants, and it benefits future readers by ensuring that current readers are satisfied and, if not, that their comments and opinions are heard and taken into account. Your opinions count!

1 Why did you purchase *Breast Sonography Review*? (Circle primary reason.)

 REGISTRY REVIEW   COURSE TEXT   CLINICAL REFERENCE   CME ACTIVITY

2 Have you used *Breast Sonography Review* for other reasons, too? (Circle all that apply.)

 REGISTRY REVIEW   COURSE TEXT   CLINICAL REFERENCE   CME ACTIVITY

3 To what extent did *Breast Sonography Review* meet its stated objectives and your needs? (Circle one.)

 GREATLY   MODERATELY   MINIMALLY   INSIGNIFICANTLY

4 The content of *Breast Sonography Review* was (circle one):

 JUST RIGHT   TOO BASIC   TOO ADVANCED

5 The quality of the questions and explanations was mainly (circle one):

 EXCELLENT   GOOD   FAIR   POOR

6 The manner in which *Breast Sonography Review* presents the material is mainly (circle one):

 EXCELLENT   GOOD   FAIR   POOR

7 If you used this book to prepare for the registry exam, did you also use other materials or take any exam-preparation courses?

 NO   YES (PLEASE SPECIFY WHAT MATERIALS AND COURSES)

 _____
 _____
 _____

8 If you used this book for a course, please name the course, the instructor's name, the name of the school or program, and any other textbooks you may have used:

 COURSE/INSTRUCTOR/SCHOOL OR PROGRAM:

 _____
 _____
 _____

OTHER TEXTBOOKS:

_____
_____
_____

9   What did you like best about *Breast Sonography Review*?

_____
_____
_____
_____

10 What did you like least about *Breast Sonography Review*?

_____
_____
_____
_____

11 If you used *Breast Sonography Review* to prepare for the ARDMS exam in the Breast, did you pass?

YES   NO   HAVEN'T YET TAKEN IT

12 May we quote any of your comments in our catalogs or promotional material?

YES   NO   FURTHER COMMENT . . .

_____
_____
_____
_____
_____
_____
_____
_____
_____
_____
_____
_____

CME QUIZ

Please answer the following questions after you have completed the CME activity. There is one <u>best</u> answer for each question. Circle it on the answer sheet. The passing criterion is 70%. The applicant can make no more than 3 attempts to pass and earn credit.

1. The term for rapid breast enlargement at puberty is:

   A. Gynecomastia
   B. Menarche
   C. Hyperplasia
   D. Thelarche
   E. Athelia

2. Your patient presents with skin thickening. Which of the following causes of this condition is NOT benign?

   A. Irradiation
   B. Lymphatic obstruction
   C. Nephritic syndrome
   D. Mastitis
   E. Heart failure

3. Polymastia most commonly occurs in the following location:

   A. Facial
   B. Nuchal
   C. Periumbilical
   D. Mediastinal
   E. Axillary

4. The noninvasive type of cancer that causes ductal distention filled with cheese-like material and calcifications is the:

   A. Phyllodes tumor
   B. Lobular carcinoma in situ
   C. Non-comedo type
   D. Comedo type
   E. Medullary carcinoma

5. The term for breast tissue that extends into the axilla is:

   A. Tail of Spence
   B. Mastos fascia
   C. Premammary zone
   D. The colostrum
   E. Montgomery's zone

6. Which of the following conditions can NOT mimic cancer?

   A. Sclerosing adenosis

   B. Galactocele
   C. Fat necrosis
   D. Diabetic mastopathy
   E. Radial scar

7. What is the term for the smallest functional unit of the glandular breast tissue?

   A. Ductule
   B. Lobule
   C. Acini
   D. Intralobular terminal duct
   E. Extralobular terminal duct

8. Each female breast usually contains how many lobes?

   A. 30–40
   B. 1–5
   C. 10–15
   D. 5–10
   E. 15–20

9. Why are standoff pads thicker than 1 cm NOT recommended?

   A. They affect the optimal placement of the fixed elevation plane focus.
   B. They cause decreased penetration and an inability to see the chest wall.
   C. They cause enhancement of echoes in the mammary zone.
   D. They make the skin line look thicker than normal.
   E. They compress the mammary layer and make it look fibrotic.

10. Which of the following is NOT considered a sonographic feature of malignancy?

   A. Taller than wide
   B. Spiculation
   C. Angular margins
   D. Enhancement
   E. Markedly hypoechoic

11. All of the following statements are correct EXCEPT:

   A. Skin is hyperechoic compared to fat.
   B. Cooper's ligaments are isoechoic compared to fat.
   C. Fat exhibits a medium shade of gray.
   D. Muscle is hypoechoic compared to fat.
   E. Fibroglandular tissue is hyperechoic compared to fat.

12. The following characteristic is considered a variation of spiculation:

   A. Thick echogenic halo
   B. Disruption of tissue planes
   C. Microlobulation
   D. Duct extension
   E. Angular margins

13. Your patient presents with a bloody nipple discharge. Which benign mass can cause this condition?

   A. Fibroma
   B. Papilloma
   C. Lipoma
   D. Cyst
   E. Hamartoma

14. What is the term for the lymph nodes located between the pectoral muscles?

   A. Infraclavicular nodes
   B. Intrapectoral nodes
   C. Axillary nodes
   D. Rotter's nodes
   E. Parasternal nodes

15. All of the following are considered true cancers EXCEPT:

   A. Comedo type
   B. Lobular carcinoma in situ
   C. Ductal carcinoma in situ
   D. Medullary
   E. Papillary

16. Which of the following diagnostic modalities is used for ductography?

   A. Nuclear medicine
   B. Sonography
   C. Computerized tomography
   D. Magnetic resonance imaging
   E. Mammography

17. This finding would NOT be a reliable diagnostic indicator for malignancy:

   A. Overall acoustic shadowing
   B. Posterior enhancement
   C. Incompressibility
   D. Positive color flow
   E. Hypoechogenicity

18. The echogenicity of all tissues of the breast is most similar to that of:

    A. Fascia
    B. Glandular parenchyma
    C. Fat
    D. Muscle
    E. Ligaments

19. This malignant breast tumor is considered noninvasive:

    A. Ductal carcinoma in situ
    B. Medullary
    C. Inflammatory carcinoma
    D. Metastatic breast cancer
    E. All of the above

20. The procedure that carries the best chance for tumor localization is:

    A. Large-core biopsy
    B. Spring-loaded core biopsy
    C. FNAB
    D. Advanced breast biopsy instrumentation (ABBI)
    E. Vacuum-assisted mammotomy

21. Which implant site lowers the risk of capsular contracture?

    A. Submuscular
    B. Subcutaneous
    C. Prepectoral
    D. Intramammary
    E. Submammary

22. When mastitis is associated with lactation it is referred to as:

    A. Ectatic
    B. Periductal
    C. Puerperal
    D. Granulomatous
    E. Apocrine

23. In what subgroup of the population are fibroadenomas more common?

    A. Hispanics
    B. African Americans
    C. Asians
    D. Caucasians
    E. Ethnicity is irrelevant

24. What type of cells line the inner portion of the breast ducts?

    A. Cuboidal
    B. Transitional
    C. Basal
    D. Epithelial
    E. Squamous

25. The following annotation method for breast imaging is considered appropriate:

    A. 123-ABC
    B. Clock-face
    C. Side/quadrant
    D. None of the above
    E. All of the above

26. Which of the following is NOT a secondary diagnostic feature?

    A. Skin changes
    B. Interruption of tissue planes
    C. Lymph node enlargement
    D. Homogenicity
    E. Tumor extension

27. The benign pathology known as the "swiss cheese disease," because of its sonographic appearance, is:

    A. Fibroadenoma
    B. Mondor's disease
    C. Phyllodes tumor
    D. Fibrocystic dysplasia
    E. Juvenile papillomatosis

28. This breast cancer can mimic a fibroadenoma:

    A. Medullary
    B. Papillary
    C. Invasive ductal
    D. Colloid
    E. Tubular

29. All of the following statements suggest that a mass is benign EXCEPT:

    A. The mass is hyperechoic.
    B. The mass has microlobulations.
    C. The mass shows acoustic enhancement.
    D. The mass is horizontal.
    E. The mass has a thin pseudocapsule.

30. For which breast imaging modality is gadolinium used as a contrast agent?

   A. Nuclear medicine
   B. Sonography
   C. Mammography
   D. Magnetic resonance imaging
   E. Computerized tomography

31. Which of these statements would NOT suggest malignancy?

   A. A mass is incompressible.
   B. A mass is non-parallel to the chest wall.
   C. A mass has irregular, ill-defined margins.
   D. A mass is markedly hypoechoic.
   E. A mass has 2–3 macrolobulations.

32. The characteristic appearance of an intracapsular silicone rupture is known as the:

   A. Wavy line sign
   B. Stepladder sign
   C. Noose sign
   D. Teardrop sign
   E. Linguini sign

33. Which of these sonographic findings is NOT characteristic of a complex cyst?

   A. Intramural nodule
   B. Fluid debris level
   C. Septations
   D. Wall thickening
   E. Oval shape

34. Which of these procedures can help differentiate benign from malignant masses when sonography is inconclusive?

   A. Galactography
   B. Ductography
   C. Magnetic resonance imaging
   D. Nuclear medicine
   E. Sentinel node procedure

35. Which of the following factors does NOT increase the brightness of echoes?

   A. Dynamic range
   B. Transducer frequency
   C. Overall gain
   D. TGC

E. Power output

36. Which of the following is the most common silicone breast implant?

   A. Double lumen, outer silicone, and inner saline
   B. Double lumen saline
   C. Double lumen, outer saline, and inner silicone
   D. Single lumen, gel-filled
   E. Direct silicone injection

37. Where is lateral resolution best?

   A. Fraunhofer zone
   B. Fresnel zone
   C. Transmit zone
   D. Focal zone
   E. Near zone

38. All of the following might be considered complications of breast trauma EXCEPT:

   A. Skin thickening
   B. Hamartoma
   C. Hematoma
   D. Fat necrosis
   E. Scarring

39. Which of the following masses would NOT require biopsy or aspiration?

   A. Solid irregular lesion
   B. Enlarged irregular lymph node
   C. Nontender small simple cyst
   D. Large painful cyst
   E. Irregular complex mass

40. Increased intensity of echoes beneath a structure is called:

   A. Enhancement
   B. Reflection
   C. Shadowing
   D. Refraction
   E. Reverberation

41. All of the following statements are true EXCEPT:

   A. Advanced breast biopsy instrumentation (ABBI) can completely excise small lesions.
   B. Mammotomy can completely excise small lesions.
   C. Fine-needle aspiration provides tissues for cytologic analysis.
   D. Histologic analysis is more conclusive than cytologic analysis.

E. Cytologic analysis is more conclusive than histologic analysis.

42. When the overall gain control is increased:

   A. Artifactual echoes are produced.
   B. Gray scale is increased.
   C. Penetration is reduced.
   D. Penetration is increased.
   E. Frame rate is reduced.

43. AIUM standards indicate that all of the following information should be indicated on sonography images of the breast EXCEPT:

   A. Facility name
   B. Date
   C. Patient's age
   D. Patient's social security number
   E. Patient's name/ID #

44. All of the following are sonographic characteristics of a simple cystic mass EXCEPT:

   A. Thin walls
   B. Posterior enhancement
   C. Anechoic
   D. Shadowing
   E. Sharply marginated

45. When you decrease depth:

   A. Depth penetration improves.
   B. Frame rate increases.
   C. The frequency of sound used increases.
   D. Gray scale is increased.
   E. The sound intensity decreases.

46. Mammographic stereotactic guidance is required for:

   A. Vacuum-assisted mammotomy
   B. Advanced breast biopsy instrumentation (ABBI)
   C. Spring-loaded core biopsy
   D. Fine-needle aspiration biopsy (FNAB)
   E. None of the above

47. When you select multiple focal zones, you:

   A. Increase penetration
   B. Increase frequency
   C. Decrease frequency
   D. Increase frame rate
   E. Decrease frame rate

48. The colloid carcinoma is also known as:

    A. Mucinous
    B. Metaplasia
    C. Cystosarcoma phyllodes
    D. Sarcoma
    E. Papillomatosis

49. The marker on mammograms will always be seen in the region toward the:

    A. Medial breast
    B. Top of the film
    C. Axilla
    D. Nipple
    E. Bottom of the film

50. This sonographic feature would be considered benign:

    A. Microlobulations
    B. Angular margins
    C. Marked hypoechogenicity
    D. Marked hyperechogenicity
    E. Thick capsule

51. Which organization developed the BI-RADS Classification for Mammography and Sonography?

    A. ACR
    B. SDMS
    C. AMA
    D. AIUM
    E. None of the above

52. Identify the statement that is FALSE:

    A. Cancers usually show more internal blood flow.
    B. Some cancers show posterior enhancement.
    C. Abscess and hematomas can disrupt tissue planes.
    D. Microcalcifications can be seen in benign and malignant tumors.
    E. All cancers show some degree of shadowing.

53. When the long axis of a mass is parallel to the skin line, the mass is:

    A. Ductal in origin
    B. Taller than wide
    C. Wider than tall
    D. Probably malignant
    E. Superficial

54. The following mass can develop secondary to traumatic fat necrosis:

    A. Milk cyst
    B. Seroma
    C. Oil cyst
    D. Simple cyst
    E. Sebaceous cyst

55. BI-RADS classification Category 2 indicates:

    A. Suspicious abnormality
    B. Benign finding
    C. Inconclusive
    D. Negative
    E. Probably benign

56. Which of the following features concerning nipple discharge would NOT be considered benign?

    A. Multiple duct orifices
    B. Green, milky discharge
    C. Expressible only discharge
    D. Bilateral
    E. Clear discharge

57. Your 25-year-old patient presents with a solid breast mass. The most common solid mass found in women younger than 30 years of age is the:

    A. Fibroadenoma
    B. Invasive ductal carcinoma
    C. Medullary carcinoma
    D. Papilloma
    E. Phyllodes tumor

58. Which feature would suggest lymph node pathology?

    A. Hilar blood flow from single artery
    B. Thin capsule
    C. Central fatty hilum
    D. Hypoechoic cortex
    E. Round shape

59. Your patient has developed a clear fluid-filled mass following surgery. She most likely has a/an:

    A. Hematoma
    B. Oil cyst
    C. Seroma
    D. Galactocele
    E. Cyst

60. The malignant counterpart of the benign fibroadenoma is the:

   A. Phyllodes
   B. Invasive ductal
   C. Medullary
   D. Colloid
   E. Lobular

PART 11

Exam Outline

The American Registry of Diagnostic Medical Sonographers publishes its exam outlines and other important information on its website (www.ARDMS.org). Visit the site for complete and current information about applying for and taking the registry examinations.

The outline for each exam indicates the approximate percentage of the exam that a particular topic represents. This information is important because it indicates the relative importance of each topic and allows you to study more effectively. For example, anatomy and physiology questions represent 18% of the Breast exam, whereas patient care questions represent 5%.

The outline for the Breast specialty examination appears below.

I. **Anatomy and Physiology (18%)**
   A. Normal anatomy and physiology
   B. Perfusion and function

II. **Pathology (30%)**
   A. Abnormal perfusion and function
   B. Benign vs. suspicious

III. **Patient Care (5%)**
   A. Communications

IV. **Integration of Data (15%)**
   A. Incorporate outside data (Clinical assessment, Health & Physical [H&P], Lab values)
   B. Reporting results

V. **Protocols (4%)**
   A. Clinical standards and guidelines
   B. Measurement techniques

VI. Physics (9%)

A. Artifacts
B. Hemodynamics
C. Imaging instruments

VII. Treatment (12%)

A. Interventional procedures
B. Intraoperative procedures
C. Sonographer role in procedures

VIII. Other (7%)

A. New technologies